ALSO BY ALBERT ROSENFELD

The Quintessence of Irving Langmuir
The Second Genesis: The Coming Control of Life

PROLONGEVITY

Pro longevity

*A report
on the scientific
discoveries now being made about aging
and dying, and their promise of
an extended human life span—
without old age.*

ALBERT ROSENFELD

Alfred A. Knopf NEW YORK 1976

THIS IS A BORZOI BOOK
PUBLISHED BY ALFRED A. KNOPF, INC.

Since this page cannot legibly accommodate all permissions
acknowledgments, they may be found on pages v and vi.

Library of Congress Cataloging in Publication Data
Rosenfeld, Albert.
Prolongevity.
Bibliography: p.
Includes index.
1. Longevity. 2. Aging. I. Title.
QP85.R65   612.6'7   76–13705
ISBN 0–394–48929–2

Manufactured in the United States of America
First Edition

For my wife,
Lillian,
after twenty-eight years.

Looking forward
to the next twenty-eight.

Acknowledgments

Gerontology, the scientific study of the aging process, is one of the most important frontier areas in current biomedical research. As a science journalist, I have been following its erratic progress with great fascination for a number of years, and the time seems ripe for a popular synthesis—not an attempt to describe, in exhaustive detail, an entire science, but rather an exploration of the most recent developments, experiments, and theories that might serve as combined reportage, interpretation, and responsible speculation. I have tried to keep the reportage as clear and accurate as possible, and to separate it from what is purely interpretative and speculative. To undertake such a task, especially in an area where there is little consensus among the credentialed experts, requires a certain presumptuousness; but without a willingness to presume, very little science would ever be written for the public. I have done a great deal of homework over a long period of time and have sought the advice and instruction of many of the leading investigators in gerontology and related areas of biology—who do often disagree with one another, as will be apparent in the course of this book.

I am of course deeply indebted to those whose writings I have studied; but I want to extend my particular thanks to the people who have generously and cheerfully granted personal interviews; allowed me to visit their offices, homes, and laboratories; answered my phone calls and letters, and referred me to other valuable sources of information. In some cases the communication amounted to no more than a single conversation or exchange of correspondence; in others, it entailed hours and even days at a time of intensive talk and shared speculation, as well as subsequent communications and revisits in order to clarify points of confusion or to give one investigator the opportunity to respond to a challenge raised by another.

I shall not attempt to list my numerous benefactors—though most of them will appear somewhere in the pages of the book, or at least in a bibliographical mention. For one thing, it is difficult to express degrees of gratitude where it is not really measurable; for another, I would not want anyone to be blamed for the views expressed here—unless a given view is clearly attributed to a specified individual. No single one of my sources or mentors was given the opportunity to read this book in its entirety prior to publication. The responsibility for any errors of fact or interpretation—always a risk in a work of this scope—must be borne by the author alone.

A note on style: An editorial decision was made to drop the designation "Dr." throughout the book, mainly because just about everyone mentioned is a doctor of one kind or another. As a rule, in the main text of the book, the investigator's full name and affiliation is given the first time he or she is mentioned, but usually not thereafter. Similarly, the full names of institutions are often abbreviated on repetition; thus, for example, the Gerontological Research Center in Baltimore becomes GRC/Baltimore, the State University of New York at Buffalo becomes SUNY/Buffalo, and the University of Texas Medical Branch in Galveston becomes UTMB/Galveston.

My research required the use of a number of different libraries. My special thanks, however, are due the National Foundation–March of Dimes for providing easy access to indispensable journals and books, particularly in the area of genetics. I am deeply grateful, too, to Emil Frey, Director of the Moody Medical Library at UTMB/Galveston for permission to use the superb facilities and collections at one of the nation's very finest medical-school libraries.

One more set of thank-yous: to the *Saturday Review* for permission to use material originally gathered for, and in some cases used in, its pages; and to the *TIME-LIFE Nature/Science Annual* for similar permission to use material collected in the course of writing one of its articles.

Finally, for rendering the details of the task much easier than would otherwise have been the case, my heartfelt appreciation to

Dina Gutierrez for her typing and secretarial services, and her sharp eye for the author's typos.

And, of course, to Lillian, for putting up with it all for so long.

—A.R.

New Rochelle, N.Y.

1976

Contents

Preface

"Every day you get older—that's a law"

—Butch Cassidy to the Sundance Kid

Built into the beginning of life is the end of it.

Every individual who is born into the world inevitably follows a predictable course, unless his life is cut short by accident or disease. He develops to maturity, remains at a productive plateau for a given number of years, then gradually declines, ages, dies.

I say "inevitably" because this is what has always happened to every human being who has lived on earth. A conspicuous minority remain vigorous longer than others, some notable random examples from recent history being Bertrand Russell, George Bernard Shaw, Margaret Sanger, Winston Churchill, Albert Schweitzer, Marianne Moore, Pablo Picasso, Grandma Moses, Konrad Adenauer, Wanda Landowska, Georgia O'Keeffe, Pablo Casals—men and women who remained creative and productive into their eighties and nineties. Others seem not only to remain vigorous in their later years, but to live out a longer lifetime. Pockets of impressive longevity have been reported (though the reports have not been universally accepted as factual) in the Soviet Republic of Georgia, in the Himalayan heights of Hunza in Kashmir, and among the Andean Indians of the Vilcabamba Valley in Ecuador. In all these places, quantities of hardy individuals claim to have survived well past the century mark.

Even in the United States, where 10 per cent of the population is now over sixty-five, some 13,000 men and women are more than a hundred years old. Of those over sixty-five, 86 per cent are afflicted with one or more of the chronic degenerative diseases. But few observers emphasize the reverse side of these statistics: 14 per cent do *not* have these diseases. Though all old people eventually fall prey to deteriorative changes, many seem to escape the major ravages of aging until they are very old indeed. Why is it that one man is bald and toothless twenty years sooner than his next-door neighbor? Is his neighbor just lucky, or is long life somehow written into his genes?

Some animals are unusually long-lived. The Galapagos tortoise, for instance, can go on for well over 150 years, perhaps even live into the beginning of a third century. Some trees of the arid American West are believed to have endured for hundreds, even thousands, of years. In the mid-1950's, Edmund Schulman of the University of Arizona's pioneering Laboratory of Tree Ring Research began finding bristlecone pines in California that were nearly a thousand years older than the oldest known sequoias—until then rated the most ancient living things on earth. In 1957, Schulman—only a year before his own death at the age of forty-nine—discovered a bristlecone pine nearly 5,000 years old, with its tree-ring data going back to the time of Nineveh and Babylon. In the "childhood" of that tree, the Pyramids were just being built.

It is possible that someone may yet turn up a living organism that predates even this Methuselah of the plant world, perhaps some bacterium that has remained frozen under the polar icecap. But we know of no organism which has lived forever—no person, no animal, no plant. Yet there exists in every living organism an essential component that does appear to "live forever." It is DNA, deoxyribonucleic acid, which maintains headquarters in the nucleus of each living cell. With its celebrated "double helix" architecture, DNA is the master molecule of heredity—in fact, of all life. It is what the chromosomes and their constituent genes are made of. DNA is the molecule from which all life on earth seems to have sprung, from its dawn in prehistory through all the millennia of evolution, from protozoa to dinosaurs to people, all of whose "genetic codes" have been surprisingly alike.

DNA is millions and millions of years old—yet shows no signs of old age. As far as we know, DNA is the only organic substance in the universe that possesses the information to ensure its own virtual immortality. DNA has the unique ability to duplicate itself, again and again, almost without limit, as long as there are materials around from which it can manufacture new copies of itself. Following the genetic manual of instructions that is encoded biochemically into its molecular structure, it knows how to take what it needs from the environment and put it together as more DNA—as well as more of the other things it needs, such as proteins, to keep alive the body which it inhabits.

In the normal pattern of our lives, we mature, we marry, have children, grow old, and die. The DNA in our cells may grow old along with us (at least, we believe it does), but it maintains its immortality—though occasionally changing some of its characteristics—by renewing itself in the mother's egg and the father's sperm. These combine to create a new individual who will carry on, unbroken, the chain of human life.

It is as if DNA *used* us to keep *itself* going. It discards individuals as blithely as a snake sheds its successive skins after they have outlived their usefulness, and simply continues its own life in the next generation. We like to think that *we* use DNA, that it is our way—or nature's, or God's—of perpetuating the human race. One might just as readily speculate that the purpose of human life is to perpetuate DNA!

We do take it as natural law that the outcome of every lived-out life must be aging and degeneration as precursors of death. But scientists have demonstrated in the past that even natural laws are subject to human amendment, once we learn how they work. Now that we have begun to fathom DNA's game perhaps we can learn, by manipulating the genetic information, to use our new knowledge to gain some measure of immortality for ourselves—to use DNA rather than permit ourselves to continue to be used, passively resigned to our "fate," by it.

Every species of multicellular organism seems to have a fixed life span, but "fixed" under usual circumstances does not necessarily mean immutable under all circumstances. In fact, a number of experiments in recent years have suggested convincingly that there is nothing absolute about life's preordained endpoint in time. And this conviction has come about through the use of relatively crude techniques that are a long way from the sophisticated control implied in schemes for manipulating the DNA.

If you restrict the diet of rats during early development, for example, to almost a semi-starvation (though still nutritious) level, you extend their life spans. If you hook an old rat up to a younger one by a surgical procedure called parabiosis, so that the two share a common blood circulation as Siamese twins do, the older rat lives considerably longer than his unhooked-up littermates. An old cockroach, similarly hooked up by parabiosis to a young roach, will regain its youthful capacity to regenerate severed limbs. If you feed antioxidant compounds to mice or suppress the activity of their immune systems in certain circumstances, you retard the rate of aging. If you lower the temperature of certain cold-blooded creatures by a few degrees, they live longer. A combination of cooling and diet restriction at different periods of its development will triple the life span of the microscopic water-dwelling rotifer.

If you transplant skin cells from an aging animal to a younger one of the same species; then, as that one ages, retransplant the skin to another young one; and so on in serial fashion, the transplanted cells will outlive their original donor by a wide margin. If you add certain ingredients to the culture medium of human cells in tissue culture, they will live longer than they normally would—"normally" in this instance referring to the usual artificial conditions of life in laboratory tissue cultures.

There is a rare childhood disease called progeria in which the victim, afflicted by an accelerated aging process, shows many signs of premature senescence in early childhood and dies of apparent old age in his early teens. If the aging process can thus be speeded up by accident, can it perhaps be slowed down by design?

All very fascinating, but rats, roaches, and rotifers aren't people.

And isolated cells in tissue culture are not the same as whole living organisms.

And the course of a rare disease is not necessarily related in any way to what happens in the normal aging process.

And there is no unanimity among the experts as to what causes aging and what, if anything, might be done about it. In fact, someone recently commented that there seem to be as many theories about aging as there are gerontologists.

Nevertheless, there has been some noticeable convergence among theorists, and growing agreement on the kinds of research that might test the validity of their hypotheses within reasonable periods of time, at reasonable expense. Moreover, the gerontologists themselves —those scientists who specialize in the study of the aging process— show every sign of mounting optimism and excitement as they pursue their far-flung investigations.

This book, as it surveys current gerontological research and theory, will explore the obvious questions about the prospects of slowing down or even abolishing old age, and of significantly extending the vigorous years of our lives. The central question, of course, is whether or not we can really hope to do it. If that answer is affirmative, we will then have to examine the ethical question implied by the new biological possibilities—whether we *should* proceed to do it, just because we can. And we will want to make some guesses as to when we might expect the advances to occur, as well as what the consequences might be—personal, national, global—when the new knowledge begins to be acquired and applied.

Any consideration of consequences must of course be classified as sheer academic speculation unless the plausibility of success can first be reasonably documented. Hence the largest portion of the book will be addressed to that first crucial question: whether or not we can feasibly hope to succeed.

The subject of gerontology is vast and complex, and in such constant flux that it cannot be fixed in place like an insect embedded in amber, with all details known and visible, but must rather be described in flight. Moreover, there is still much disagreement among the creators of the new knowledge, who often challenge one another's facts and observations, as well as their interpretation of those facts and observations. Nevertheless, they do so with an air of good cheer, confident that the situation is only temporary. Gerontologists of all schools can see ahead to the time when the kind of facts they can all agree upon will be in hand. Whichever theories of aging turned out to be correct, all hold out high hopes that the knowledge will contain the remedies.

The first advances will be only partial. But each significant advance should accelerate the acquisition of further knowledge and understanding. Eventually we will harness DNA and its genetic code to our own ends. When we have begun to do that, it is likely—for reasons shortly to be spelled out—that we will be well on our way to the final conquest of old age. Long before we arrive at that stage of know-how, however, even relatively modest initial successes could be significant in terms of the good years of each individual's personal life.

—A.R.
New Rochelle, N.Y.
1976

PART ONE: CAN WE DO IT?

"*It should be
the function of medicine
to have people die young
as late as possible.*"

—Ernst L. Wynder
Epidemiologist
President of the American
Health Foundation

Chapter I

THE GERONTOLOGIST
AS CAPTAIN AHAB

"Living things," according to the distinguished British zoologist J. Z. Young, of the University of London, "act as they do because they are so organized as to take actions that prevent their dissolution into the surroundings." This is especially true of those highly developed living things called people who, moved by psychology as well as biology, are equipped not only to observe but also to worry about the early signs of their dissolution into the surroundings. So moved and so equipped, they put forth great efforts—and encourage the medical profession to do the same on their behalf—to remain intact and keep their surroundings out where they belong.

Most of us, I think, believe intuitively that nature is on our side in these efforts. If only we would behave in accordance with nature's designs, assuming we could discern them, then all would surely go well with us. Indeed many sages, ancient and modern alike, have equated good health with "living in harmony with nature," an outlook they have prescribed as guide and governor of our everyday lives. In this implied scheme of things, a benevolent nature designs the human organism to go on as long as possible—perhaps forever; but the wear and tear of our days and years, augmented by our own follies, gradually slows us down and eventually does us in.

Is this an accurate portrayal of nature's game? Or has nature rather served its own purposes by *programming* us to run down and die by means of a pre-set "clock of aging"? It begins to look as if, in the matter of individual longevity, nature may not be on our side after all. At least, more and more gerontologists are coming round to the view that we are programmed to die, that the end of

3

life really *is* built, genetically, into its beginning. But this realization, if it is a true one, doesn't lead them to despair. On the contrary, it provides grounds for hope.

"Aging and death do seem to be what nature has planned for us," gerontologist Bernard L. Strehler, of the University of Southern California, readily agrees. "But what if we have other plans?" Strehler makes it plain that *he,* for one, has other plans. He characterizes death as a kind of Moby Dick, a tough, remorseless leviathan —never before conquered, to be sure, but conquerable nevertheless —and himself as one of the numerous Captain Ahabs out to get the great white whale. "And sooner or later," he vows, "we *are* going to get him!" He sounds both convinced and convincing as he plants his feet firmly on deck (he is actually standing, as he speaks, on the decklike wooden porch of his home in Agoura, California), looking every centimeter the tall, ruddy shipmaster, his eyes fixed on a far horizon. (In this case, the actual horizon—Malibu Lake's— is close at hand; and the ruddiness of Strehler's countenance is due more to a slight though chronic elevation in blood pressure than to the weathering effects of sun and wind.)

"I really hate death," he says, as we move back into the house. It is a straight-faced remark. He speaks with no trace of irony or resignation but rather in the testy, indignant tone one might use to complain about, say, air pollution, or graft at City Hall. "Death may be in accord with nature's plan *so far*. But there is no absolute principle in nature," he declares flatly, "which dictates that individual living things cannot live for indefinitely long periods of time in optimum health.

"I first became aware of death, with some sense of how unfair and how irrevocable it is, when the minister of our church died," he recalls. "I was not quite five years old when that happened." Young Bernie had already gone to bed that evening when he heard his parents crying in the living room. He went halfway down the stairs, sat for a moment in puzzlement, then asked, "Why are you crying?"

"Reverend Tiersch has died," his mother told him.

Bernie was not sure what that meant, but he started crying too. His parents hastened to assure him there was no need to be sad, really, that Reverend Tiersch was a good man and had certainly now gone to heaven to join Jesus. We all die sooner or later, they told him, and the upright minister now had a much better life to look forward to than was available on earth. Bernie, still sniffling, went back to bed thinking: If death is such a great thing for the minister, why are they still crying?

Strehler handed me a few Xeroxed pages out of a book published in 1943. They contain an essay called "Immortality," written by himself at the age of seventeen when, as a student at Central High School in Johnstown, Pennsylvania, he was awarded a Westinghouse Science Scholarship. "Immortality—that magic word is, I believe, the key to the direction which will be taken in the next great step forward in science," the essay begins. "From time immemorial man has sought, without avail, a way to eliminate or reverse the effects of time on the human body . . ."

It goes on to speak of a "protoplasmic desire for unending existence." Art and religion, literature, music, and philosophy "are all, whether so intended or not, the mediums by which we propagate our personalities and ourselves," resulting in a kind of "thought immortality." But this kind of vicarious immortality, lived through the awareness of posterity, "is not enough for man, for the innate property of protoplasm, self preservation, must be satisfied. Man will never be contented until he conquers death." After a quick survey of some of the relatively sparse gerontological data which existed in the early 1940's, the final paragraph reads: "From this and other data I have come to the conclusion that senility and death are not the inevitable ends of human existence, either as individuals or as a race, and that through scientific research we shall eventually be able to remove the sorrows of death from the human mind."

A remarkable essay for a seventeen-year-old. And here is Strehler, more than thirty years later, still talking the same way. There have been a few doubts along the way, but, by and large, he has held on to his dream. The mere fact that he has done so does not, of course, guarantee its validity. Some of his detractors might interpret Strehler's adherence to his teen-age vision as a simple failure to out-grow his adolescence. But it would be a mistake to conclude that Strehler is no less deluded in his quest than, say, Ponce de León hunting for the Fountain of Youth, or some alchemist seeking to brew an "elixir of life." His declarations may sound outlandish, but he feels he has good grounds for making them.

His grounds lie simply in the tools of biology, and in the rapidly proliferating knowledge of the basic processes of life, including human life. Strehler has done pathbreaking work of his own in gerontology, some of which will be described presently; he has written a first-rate book on the subject, *Time, Cells and Aging* (though much has happened since its publication in 1962); and had President Richard Nixon not vetoed the bill that would have established a National Institute on Aging in 1972, Strehler would certainly have been one of the candidates for its directorship. The research he has carried out, along with the mass of new information provided by numerous other investigators in the intervening years, has only served to confirm and strengthen Strehler's early optimism.

Moreover, he is far from alone in his views. A growing number of his colleagues—many of whom have expressed themselves quite independently of Strehler, and perhaps even prior to him—are now willing to countenance the belief that to grow old physiologically, merely because the calendar has marked the passage of sixty, eighty, or even one hundred years, may not, after all, be an inevitable consequence of human life. Many believe, further, that we contain within ourselves a mechanism, an elusive clock of aging whose working secrets are no longer necessarily beyond our understanding, or beyond our tampering.

These were the considerations that led the writer Alan Harrington to declare, in *The Immortalist,* "Death is an imposition on the human race, and no longer acceptable." Similar pronouncements, made in earlier centuries—such as John Donne's "Death, thou shalt die"— could only be cries of defiance. The same was still true in our own time. Dylan Thomas exhorted his father: "Do not go gentle into that good night./ Rage, rage against the dying of the light." To which Alan Harrington responds: " 'Do not go gentle into that good night' does not apply here. Rather aim not to go at all; mobilize the scientists, spend the money, and hunt death down like an outlaw."

That exhortation of Harrington's fairly describes Strehler's aims: to mobilize the scientists, spend the money, and hunt death down like an outlaw. He has been reinforced in his determination by further events in his personal life, not least of which was the death of a small daughter by drowning.

Strehler, having long since recruited himself for the effort, has spent a lot of time and energy propagandizing for the cause, particularly among fellow scientists. Other gerontologists, whom we will meet in due course, have been similarly self-mobilizing as well as evangelistic. The job has not been easy. "Gerontology," as Strehler has lamented, "used to be too frequently associated in people's minds with quacks and dubious rejuvenators. It was considered a not quite respectable branch of biology to choose as a career." (As he said that, I remembered a British geneticist telling me that gerontologists were, by and large, "a ragbag lot.") But investigators with unassailable credentials have continued to move into the field. And now that the United States has officially established a National Institute on Aging in 1974 as part of the National Institutes of Health, new people may be lured to where the money is.

"Who has not felt a nostalgic or desperate longing to see the 'I' perpetuated in some form," Strehler has written, in *Perspectives in Biology and Medicine,* "to live beyond the pale of what we know as real?" Later in the same series of sketches, Strehler—who yearns for prolongevity in the same shameless, articulate manner as ever did the late Miguel de Unamuno—bursts into poetry:

> Do men truly, truly go to dust and speak no more
> When breathing stops?

And again:

> Time (Oh, Time) I curse your ugly hours
> And would wring a respite
> From your bloodless pursing lips!

Bernie Strehler smokes too much. And, midway down his long athletic frame, a paunch has become visible. When his friends chide him for not taking better care of himself (he knows he should) and working too hard (he knows he does), he smiles and—ever-mindful of himself as Ahab, and Death as the Great White Whale—replies, "Maybe I'll get him before he gets me."

Few gerontologists, even among the avant garde which Strehler symbolizes, would predict the outright abolition of death. But many would certainly go along with the more modest forecast that old age, with all its attendant aches and ills, may well be abolished and the life span extended, perhaps for a substantial number of years.

Chapter II

SENESCENCE AS A CURABLE DISEASE

Gerontologists take pains to emphasize that they are not practitioners of the medical specialty of *geriatrics,* which concerns itself primarily with the study and treatment of old people's diseases. Gerontology (*gerōn* is Greek for old man) seeks rather to prevent people from getting old at all. It studies the aging process itself, and in *all* species.

The two areas do overlap, of course, especially since an increasing number of gerontologists are finding it useful to take a somewhat geriatric view of the matter—that old age itself is just another disease. It is a disease everyone gets, to be sure, and the individual who survives all the other diseases invariably succumbs to this one. But just because a disease is universal and has always been fatal does not, in this revised reasoning, make it inevitably so. Merely to think about aging as a degenerative ailment, rather than as man's eternal and preordained fate, is to put it in the category of a medical problem— something your doctor may some day hope to do something about.

Another way of expressing one of gerontology's unabashed aims, then, is: to cure or prevent the disease we now call old age, or senescence. Its other major aim—to extend the human life span—is puzzling to many people who, aware that we already do live a lot longer than we used to, ask: Haven't medical scientists already extended the human life span? The answer is that they have not. What they have extended is the *average life expectancy.* We do live much longer, on the average, because we have eliminated so many of the diseases and circumstances which used to kill us off prematurely in such large numbers. But the average life *span,* the maximum longevity of the individual, has remained essentially unchanged.

In ancient Greece, for instance—let's say Athens in the age of Pericles—the average life expectancy was something like twenty-two years. But individuals did live to ripe old ages in those days too. Their number was small enough, however, to render them an elite in most ancient societies, where their seasoning was rare and their wisdom prized. They made up the powerful kosmoi of Crete, the ephors of Sparta, the archons of Athens. A Greek who reached the age of seventy in the fifth century B.C. had just as many years to live—perhaps more, since he had to be tougher to have survived so long under such conditions—as does the seventy-year-old of today, who has merely reached his average life expectancy.

Sophocles wrote *Oedipus Rex* when he was seventy-five, and won the last of his many dramatic prizes at eighty-five, still going strong. And he needed no contemporary equivalent of Masters and Johnson to tell him that men of that age were still sexually viable. He not only kept his bed and bones warm with the famous hetaira Theoris (who was succeeded at an even later date by Archippe), but also became a father again. In fact, his legitimate son, Iophon, afraid he would be disinherited in favor of Theoris or her child, tried to have his aging father declared incompetent. But Sophocles satisfied the court he was sound in mind by reading them a few choruses from the drama he was even then in the midst of composing—probably *Oedipus at Colonus,* which he finished at eighty-nine, a year before his death. This is not to say that vigorous longevity such as Sophocles' goes unmatched today—I have already cited a number of examples to the contrary—but simply that it is still rare. The maximum life span has *not* been extended. And our contemporaries who reach seventy, eighty, and ninety probably have just as many aches and failings as the ancients did, though there may be a few more medications available to ease their more troublesome pains.

The fact that so many of us do reach seventy and beyond is what makes us more aware than ever how universal are the ravages of the aging process—ravages that made even Sophocles, for all his honors and amours, a thoroughgoing pessimist in his declining years. Observing the inexorable nature of these changes, their variety, their sheer multiplicity, and their interlocking complexity, most traditional gerontologists have maintained an unshakable conservatism despite the boldness of their stated goals. The prevailing view, understandably, has been that, considering the multi-faceted nature of the aging process, it would be foolish to count on any significant progress toward final answers until countless further generations of painstaking experimentation shall have passed.

Typical of this cautious outlook, even among scientists not reputed as especially conservative, is the conclusion of a 1962 paper in *Proceedings of the Royal Society.* Its author, anatomist P. L. Krohn of the University of Birmingham, after describing a brilliantly original series of experiments designed to study the effects of transplantation on aging tissue, finally appends this demurrer: "Nothing has been said to imply that problems of old age are likely soon to be solved by this approach. . . . The solution will probably come as slowly and insidiously as the ageing process itself."

But the spirited avant garde which Strehler symbolizes is almost evangelical in its urgency, in its conviction that significant progress can be made within our own lifetimes, even within this century. How *much* progress? How significant? How soon? There is no way to forecast with precision. But the more confident gerontologists do not rule out the possibility of buying a little extra time for themselves personally while waiting for the larger advances to be accomplished —much as a leukemia victim might hope for the larger breakthroughs to occur while he is in remission.

Scientists who a few years earlier would have deplored such speculations as being in the realm of the quack and the con man are now distressed that the general public just won't give serious credence to the new possibilities. If people begin to believe in them, progress will certainly occur more rapidly. Alex Comfort is convinced not only that a project to slow down aging is feasible but that it could be carried out for relatively modest sums of money.

What worries some gerontologists more than public attitudes is the skepticism of some of their own biological colleagues, who seem to regard them somewhat pityingly, as if they were, like O'Neill's boozers in *The Iceman Cometh,* deluding themselves with wild pipedreams. Listen, for example, to Lewis Thomas, president of the Memorial Sloan-Kettering Cancer Institute and professor of pathology and medicine at the Cornell University College of Medicine, giving a major address before the American College of Surgeons in Houston on March 27, 1974: "If we are not struck down, prematurely, by one or another of today's diseases, we live a certain length of time and then we die, and I doubt that medicine will ever gain a capacity to do anything much to modify this. *I can see no reason for trying, and no hope of success anyway.* [Italics mine.] At a certain age, it is in our nature to wear out, to come unhinged and to die, and that is that." It is not that I would single out Lewis Thomas as representing the old-fogey school of biology. Quite the opposite. He is one of the more liberal and forward-looking members of the biomedical community, a man of great vision and imagination, the author of that marvelously insightful book of biophilosophical essays, *The Lives of a Cell.* Yet Lewis Thomas, in the same speech in which he decries the prevalent pessimism in other areas of biomedical research, can say of the gerontological quest in the year 1974: "I can see no reason for trying, and no hope of success anyway."*

There exists, in biomedical science (and practically everywhere else too), a phenomenon I think of as The Josh Billings Syndrome. The name derives from Billings's celebrated observation: "The trouble with people is not that they don't know, but that they know so much that ain't so." The syndrome may be defined as the collection of tendencies that lead even the most authoritative experts (in fact, *especially* the most authoritative experts) to let what they think they know get in the road of what they might learn. If they know something ain't so, it ain't hardly worth looking at—right? They forget that what they know now ain't necessarily so forever. Thus they weigh future possibilities on the basis of present knowledge, techniques, and assumptions.

I may know, for instance, how staggeringly difficult it is to carry out a certain biochemical operation to get a relatively simple piece of information. The thought of acquiring information that is incredibly more complicated, even with the most sophisticated techniques at my command (techniques which, I tend to forget, may look very crude in the light of later discoveries), seems impossibly remote, and—as a leading expert in the field—I don't mind saying so.

Thus we debate matters such as genetic engineering, the possibility that we may one day be able to manipulate our genetic material for our own purposes. This is a capacity that could be vital to any total solution to the aging problem, as you have already heard and will hear much more about in later chapters. We have, in fact, taken our first halting laboratory steps toward genetic engineering. Even so,

* This feeling was reiterated by Thomas, though not in the identical words, at a symposium held to celebrate the 75th anniversary of Rockefeller University in early 1976.

the overall problem looks so unmanageable that Nobel-calibre minds and talents such as Jacques Monod in France and Sir Macfarlane Burnet in Australia—both of whom have made impressive and original contributions to our current biological understanding—have not hesitated to predict that truly efficient genetic engineering will probably be forever beyond our grasp.

Can experts such as Monod and Burnet and Lewis Thomas— and the legion of distinguished scientists of similar persuasion—be far wrong? Yes, they can—and frequently are. Arthur C. Clarke was only half joking when he promulgated his "law" which holds that whenever an expert insists that a problem is impossible to solve, he is certainly premature and almost certainly mistaken.

As Lewis Thomas has himself written elsewhere, "The difficulties are more conspicuous when the problems are very hard and complicated and the facts not yet in. Solutions cannot be arrived at for problems of this sort until the science has been lifted through a preliminary, turbulent zone of outright astonishment. Therefore, what must be planned for, in the laboratories engaged in the work, is the totally unforeseeable. If it is centrally organized, the system must be designed primarily for the elicitation of disbelief and the celebration of surprise."

In any scientific endeavor, skepticism and caution constitute simple good sense. An eager young theorist, on fire with a Big Idea, may well be in danger of failing to consider the magnitude of the potential obstacles and, in his naïve enthusiasm, may rush ahead in the expectation that his experiments will carry him from Hello to Hallelujah in a straight line. But not many scientists, not even very young ones, sin in this direction. There is more danger that mature, experienced, eminent scientists—surer of what they know—will pronounce the goals of others as impossible, or as so remote as not to be worth the expenditure of immediate effort or attention.

It is hard to think of anything that exists in our civilized lives that would not once have been declared impossible. Look at a jumbo jet, with 350 passengers aboard. See them lifted aloft and carried across the ocean in a few hours—carried in comfort, too, fed a sumptuous meal, shown a movie, given a choice of seven stereo listening channels. That bizarre, implausible kind of occurrence does, as we know, happen routinely every day, many times a day, in many parts of the world. One would not have to go very far back in time to find the world's sanest, most knowing authorities, con-

fronted with such a description, pronouncing this kind of technological—and social—capacity to be among the more preposterous and unattainable fantasies they had ever heard.

Let's take another example, this time from the realm of pure
theoretical physics: the case of the neutrino. In 1931, studying the
distintegration phenomenon known as beta decay, Wolfgang Pauli
could account for everything except a half-unit of "spin." This was
intolerable, because it violated the law of the conservation of
angular momentum and energy. So, as an admitted "accountant's
trick" to make the atomic books balance, Pauli invented the neutrino
(Fermi's name—"little neutral one"), a most curious subatomic
"particle." Since all it possessed was that half-unit of spin, it had no
rest mass, no electrical charge, no magnetic moment, no way of
interacting with any other particle except by the most improbable
chance.

How improbable? Physicists calculated that an average neutrino
would pass through *fifty light-years of solid lead* before the chance
interaction took place. Imagine the thick lead shielding around a
nuclear reactor. Imagine it extending—the lead shield thickening,
in a solid unbroken mass—out beyond the sun, out beyond Alpha
Centauri, out as far as light could travel nonstop through the galaxy
for fifty years—and to the neutrino, all that might as well be empty
space! Trillions upon trillions of neutrinos might pass through the
earth in a split second, and no particle on earth would be the
wiser for it.

Obviously, the neutrino would always remain a purely theoretical
particle, since no one could even imagine a way by which it might
ever be detected. But then some new and unforeseen circumstances
came into being: (1) nuclear reactors, which—if neutrinos existed—
should be emitting enormous quantities of them, sufficient quantities
to increase the chance of an occasional interaction; (2) liquid
scintillating compounds, full of protons packed at unprecedented
densities, thus further increasing the chance of interactions; (3)
photomultiplier tubes, which amplify detection capabilities several
million-fold.

Now, neither nuclear reactors, scintillating compounds, nor
photomultiplier tubes were devised with the neutrino in mind. But
once they all existed, it occurred to two Los Alamos physicists,
Frederick Reines and Clyde Cowan, that they might put all those
things together for their own purposes. They did so—in a brilliantly

imaginative and painstaking series of experiments—and behold, they detected the neutrino. (They actually detected the *anti*neutrino first, but let's not complicate the story unnecessarily.) That happened in 1956, exactly twenty-five years after the invention of the particle that could never possibly be detected.

To have pronounced the neutrino forever undetectable was obviously (we now see) premature. Yet there were much better grounds for doing so than to make a similar mistake about the goals of gerontology, where one does not have to count on future technological windfalls of similar magnitude to make the search feasible, where one can already begin to envision the experimental programs that must be carried out to achieve the desired ends, and where encouraging evidence has indeed been coming in at an accelerating rate.

It is not that gerontologists of the old school—and they still undoubtedly represent the majority view—are given to making fatuously negative statements about the possibilities of success; else they would probably look for some other line of work. They simply are skeptical that any clock-of-aging theory, any genetic program, can truly encompass all the bewildering occurrences that accompany human aging: the wrinkle and sag and flab, the stoop and shuffle, the dimming and dulling of eye and ear—while, out of sight, the lungs, heart, arteries, liver, kidneys, brain, and all other organs and systems steadily slow down in function. Connective tissue gets tough and fibrous. The whole organism loses substance; it shrinks. It copes less ably with stress. It falls prey more easily to cancer, arthritis, cardiovascular disease, diabetes, autoimmune disorders, senile dementia, infection. This has always seemed to be the natural and inevitable outcome of life, and the more cautious gerontologists —though hoping for eventual success—doubt that we will be in a position to do much more about our mortal predicament for a very long time to come.

Many well-respected gerontologists, as we shall see, explain senility and death without postulating a genetic clock of aging. One such, for instance, is Robert R. Kohn of Case Western Reserve University in Cleveland, distinguished author of *Principles of Mammalian Aging*. As we sat chatting in the front lobby of the Jackson Laboratory in Bar Harbor, Maine, where we were both attending a short course in genetics, Kohn expressed the belief that the wearing down and wearing out of the organism and its parts through mere

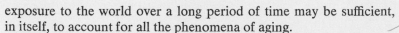

exposure to the world over a long period of time may be sufficient, in itself, to account for all the phenomena of aging.

This view is simply (perhaps over-simply) illustrated by what Sir Peter Medawar—who, among his other numerous contributions to biology, was the first to link genetics and aging—has called the "broken test-tube" theory of aging. Suppose one were to study the life experiences of a large "population" of test tubes undergoing routine use in a laboratory. Though test tubes are inanimate objects possessing no organic aging mechanisms, some might crack or break easily through some inherent structural weaknesses (birth defects?). Others would periodically be damaged or broken through chance or accident. Some of these would still be used for varying periods of time despite cracking, chipping, or corrosion. Others would be discarded and have to be replaced. Some could better withstand the strains—or would, by chance, undergo fewer strains—than others, thus would last much longer. But eventually the entire original population of test tubes will have "died" in this manner, and one could then plot a "survival curve" of aging and death. Does this not bear strong resemblances to what happens to human populations? Logical enough, admittedly. And also consistent with observations, up to a point. But far from sufficient to explain all that happens either in the laboratory or in real-life circumstances.

Because the older explanations leave so much still unexplained, interest in the avant garde view has been growing in research laboratories all over the world. This view is easy to summarize. Though even avant garde gerontologists differ in the details of their schemes and their persuasions, they are clearly coming together in the common convictions:

(1) that there does exist within ourselves an identifiable "clock of aging," a genetically determined program which dictates that we will age and die, and the rate at which this will occur;

(2) that we have an excellent chance of discovering the location (there may be more than one) of the clock of aging, as well as the nature of its operating mechanisms—and how to interfere with them to our own advantage;

(3) that, moreover, all this can begin to happen, not centuries from now, but *now,* if only the research can be carried out;

(4) that senescence may thus be started on its way to obsolescence.

Chapter III

THE GENETICS OF LIFE—
AND MAYBE DEATH

Nature does of course program us to survive. But only up to a point. That point is the production of offspring, and the rearing of those progeny to the realization of their own procreative capacities. It would appear that nature has an unflattering lack of concern for our preservation as individuals, except as instruments to ensure the perpetuation of the species. Even that may be surmising too much. So many species have come and gone in the earth's lifetime that we are well advised not to count on any guarantees, even for the human race.

What nature does seem to do, however—once a species has gone to all the evolutionary trouble of coming into being—is to give that species a fighting chance, if only through sheer extravagant multiplication. Many of the lower orders are notorious for the thousands upon thousands of eggs they produce in order that a few may survive. In fact, it is clear that *only* a few are meant to survive.

Nature is nothing if not redundant. A queen termite may, during her long reign, produce as many as 500 million eggs. Edwin Way Teale has calculated that if all the eggs generated by a single aphid in a single year were to develop into full-grown individual aphids (which are not very large creatures) and laid end to end, they would stretch for trillions of miles out into the galaxy. In our own case, nature demonstrates its prodigality by supplying the female ovary with many more thousands of oocytes than can ever ripen into eggs, while a single ejaculation of semen may release more than 250 million spermatozoa, in the hope that one may survive the journey's hazards and attain its goal. We also get plenty of chances to try

16

again, and again—a privilege not afforded the male praying mantis, for instance, whose mate bites off his head while the very act is in progress. There are many more human conceptions than there are births; we can only estimate the quantities of spontaneous abortions that occur unbeknownst to the potential parents. And of course many more babies are born than survive to the age of procreation, though our continuing intervention has now radically altered the statistics.

Nature's wildly improbable experiments with species do seem to be more random than directed, though we have far from sufficient data to arrive at such a teleological conclusion. In any case, no matter how unwieldy, inefficient, or cruel the experiment may seem in human terms—if it works, in terms of simple propagation, it tends to survive. There is a certain species of silkworm, as one example, which takes many months of development to reach the spinning stage. Once it does, it neither eats nor sleeps; all its genes are turned on to doing nothing but spinning silk for its protective cocoon. Eventually out squeezes a moth, unfolding into a creature truly beautiful to behold—who, if a mate happens along in time, copulates once, lives for a few days, and dies. All that buildup for a flickering propagative opportunity.

The Pacific salmon is a powerful orange-red fish equipped to muscle its way like a decathlon champion through all obstacles. A veritable anti-gravity machine, it swims upstream against the rapids, jumps up and over waterfalls as it moves with undistractable compulsion to its spawning grounds. Once spawning has taken place, this magnificent embodiment of strength, health, and beauty—having discharged its procreative obligations—grows old with obscene suddenness. Senility sets in virtually overnight, and, within two weeks, the great gold fish is dead.

The fate of the Pacific salmon is an extreme example of nature's loss of interest in the individual once reproduction is assured. We human individuals require more time, since our task entails more than just seeing that a mess of eggs is safely deposited and fertilized. Human children come, as a rule, one at a time. And each must be carried for many long months inside its mother, and nurtured for many long years by its parents. So the human program gives its propagators more leeway.

The individual human life may be likened to one of NASA's planetary "fly-bys"—a comparison that has grown popular in geron-

tological circles. NASA has launched many space vehicles designed
to fly by Venus, Mercury, Mars, or Jupiter. The craft's mission, in
each case, is to fly past the planet and, as it does so, with its
sophisticated array of instruments, monitors, and cameras, to pick
up and send back all possible information about the target planet's
composition, density, terrain, atmosphere, temperature gradients,
seismic activity, gravitational and magnetic fields, and whatever else
the scientists build into the experiment. The space engineers design
the vehicle and all its instruments with great care and precision. If
everything does not survive the long and dangerous trip in good
enough condition to function properly when it arrives, then the
whole effort has been wasted. So all systems are meticulously moni-
tored all the way to the planet; the data that is sent back constitutes
a treasury of new knowledge; the scientists and engineers are elated.
But when the fly-by's task is done, the designers lose all further
interest in the vehicle. They have their "baby." The vehicle may go
on out into space for a long time. Its instruments may even continue
to function for some time; but nobody cares. In some fly-bys, a self-
destruct mechanism may be installed to ensure that the vehicle's life
comes to an explosive end at a predestined moment.

It is a reasonable analogy. Unlike the planetary fly-by, however,
we are sentient vehicles, and *we* care about our individual fates,
even if the designer no longer does. Moreover, we are intelligent,
and have been accumulating sufficient knowledge about our own
workings to give us hope that we can now begin to do something to
modify what was formerly irremediable.

We have had some limited success, as already noted. In ancient
Greece, when the average life expectancy was twenty-two, that was
enough to guarantee the propagation of the species. But we have
gone on, over recent centuries, to raise this expectancy to the scrip-
tural three score and ten. Now we think we can do even better, not
only in terms of expectancy, but in extending the actual life span.
We can discover what keeps this fly-by from functioning after its
official mission is complete (by DNA's standards?); and we can
perhaps restore those functions, or prevent their running down. If
there is a self-destruct mechanism aboard—as many believe—we can
find it, and abort or dismantle it.

To understand how it is that we age and die, we must first
understand how it is that we live at all, how it is that—going against
the entropic trend, defying the Second Law of Thermodynamics

that governs the nonbiological universe, blithely increasing the complexity of its organization instead of petering out into an amorphous chaos—a single-celled organism, the original fertilized egg, guided by a compact set of genetic instructions in its nucleus, can develop into a thinking, feeling creature made up of some 60 trillion or more variegated and marvelously orchestrated living cells. The living cell, and the genetic information concentrated in its nucleus, will play a critical role in our exploration of the aging process.

But before we talk of the cell—or of the body as a population of cells—it is worth a little time and attention to dispel a widespread and mistaken impression: that the body is made *entirely* of cells, and of nothing but cells. In fact, much of the body is composed of noncellular material. "If it became possible to remove miraculously all cells from the body, as well as all free fluids," writes Macfarlane Burnet in *Genes, Dreams and Realities,* "one would have something that was still the shape of a man and probably still as difficult to disintegrate." The noncellular portions of the body are composed of the crystalline minerals that make up the bones and teeth, and the fibrous proteins—such as collagen and elastin—that constitute a large part of the body's connective tissue and help hold the bones together. All these are made up of protein molecules, and, though not cellular themselves, were originally produced by cells, and are repaired by cells—until the cells can no longer repair them. So it is still the genetic information in the cells on which their welfare and very existence depend. These fibers, these protein molecules, are all products of the same set of genetic instructions contained in the original egg.

The reason I place such emphasis on this last point is the claim occasionally raised in objection to any cellular theories of aging. If this material is not cellular, and it does age, then how can the "clock of aging" be within the cell? The answer is that, if the instructions for building and repairing these materials can be within the cell, so can the program for its aging. The contractor who built the building can also tear it down. And, so saying, let us turn to the cell itself.

The cells that make up the human body are so diverse in their sizes, shapes, functions, and what would appear to be their basic natures, that an innocent observer, examining them under the microscope, might well take them to be entirely different and unrelated species of one-celled organisms. Yet they all contain the same package of genetic information which dictates what they do, when and how they do it, and perhaps when and how they *stop* doing it.

The fertilized human egg, the initial and initiating cell, contains in its compact nucleus forty-six chromosomes. These make up a fantastically miniaturized data bank, the entire manual of genetic instructions by means of which—assuming proper food and fuel, and the absence of disastrous accidents—it will convert itself into a multi-trillion-celled adult human being. (Whether the resulting individual is to become a woman or a man is also already decided, depending on whether or not the fertilizing sperm has brought a male-producing Y chromosome to the union.) The chromosomes are composed of DNA molecules, whose spiral lattices are chemically coded with the entire individual's potential hereditary future in detail, as well as the specific information each cell needs to carry out its day-to-day operations. It has been estimated that this information, translated into English print, would fill a couple of dozen sets of the Encyclopaedia Britannica.

And, mind you, *all* this information, every detail of it, is supposed to be copied *exactly,* each time the cell divides. The presumption is that, if the individual has grown to normal maturity, every cell in his body does in fact contain the entire genetic manual—though only part of it is used.

After the first few cell divisions of embryonic life, new cells already begin to "differentiate," that is, they become a bit more specialized so that they don't need to use all the genetic information. Indeed, using it all would result in an aimless, amorphous growth rather than a patterned development, and the embryo would be spontaneously aborted. Very early in embryonic life, certain genes (a gene is the information contained on a particular segment of the DNA molecule) begin to be "switched off." They are inactivated chemically—perhaps covered up physically—by certain proteins made especially for the purpose. (These "repressors" are removed at appropriate times by "de-repressors," which thus turn the gene on again.) During embryonic and fetal development, genes are being constantly switched on and off, so that cells "know" when to divide and when to stop dividing. (Later in life, when cells lose this genetic control, they may proliferate blindly and become cancerous.)

James Bonner of Caltech has long been investigating the role of histones as the probable switch-off proteins. Now Robert T. Simpson, of NIH's National Institute of Arthritis, Metabolism and Digestive Diseases, has evidence to suggest that histones could serve as "on" switches as well. Merely by tightening up the histone *bonds,* the gene could be physically folded, almost like a pleated accordion that cannot open up to play; when the bonds are loosened, the gene's surface could once again relax, spread out, and thus be accessible—i.e., turned on. As Simpson points out, some genes may turn on only once in a lifetime, providing the blueprint needed for a specific chemical product, then turn off again forever.

At M.I.T., Nobel laureate Har Gobind Khorana, having synthesized the "tyrosine transfer RNA gene," which is found naturally in the intestinal bacterium *Escherichia coli,* is now working with his colleague Ramamoorthy Belagaje to synthesize the "stop" and "start" signals of the gene as well. When they succeed, the on-off switching devices will of course be better understood—and, once understood, perhaps eventually subject to our control.

Cells are constantly dying and being replaced during the entire prenatal period. In fact, more cells die before birth than die at death! Joan M. Whitten of Northwestern University, writing in *Science,* emphasizes the importance of cell death to the proper formation of arms, legs, fingers, and toes—or, for that matter, the limbs and digits of any vertebrate species. She reports, too, what happens to an experimental animal embryo when, at a critical point in digit formation, a chemical is injected that interferes with cell death: the digits, intended to be formed with spaces between them, grow together in webbed fashion instead. By saving the lives of the cells that were programmed to die, she crippled the animal! Such "life-saving" mistakes occur during human embryonic development and result in birth defects.

Whitten carried out experiments of her own with insects, in which embryonic cell death was believed to be much less frequent and important. But she found a "dramatic" incidence of cell death, "wholly unexpected for the insect," and concluded that "death clocks and their genetic programming seem to function in establishing shape in the insect as they do in vertebrate morphogenesis."

She then notes two contrasting types of programmed cell death. "In the vertebrate limb the death clocks function on time even when the tissue is transferred to a host of different age," which she takes as strong proof that "the timing of the vertebrate death clock is independent of external factors." When insects metamorphose from one stage to another, however, cell death is triggered from the outside—by hormones; in this case the cells are already differentiated, but have built-in receptors programmed to initiate cell death on hormonal signal.

Whitten's conclusions are concurred in by pathologist J. N. Webb, of the Edinburgh Northern Hospital Group in Scotland, who has recently been seeking the mechanisms by which cell death occurs in embryonic muscle cells. Such cell death, writes Webb in *Nature,* "takes place in a highly predictable manner and all the evidence points to it being genetically controlled." Webb believes that the programmed death of these cells "must . . . serve a function which is probably crucial to the subsequent healthy development and growth of that tissue." The failure of the death switches to operate on schedule may result in their switching on at a later time of life. This turn of events could cause a disease such as muscular dystrophy. In that case, Webb believes, the disease could be looked upon "as a normal process, but one occurring at the wrong time in the individual's life span—or else one which has not been repressed."

The course of embryonic development demands that cells of all types keep dying while new ones are created to shape the growing organism. In biology growth is not the mere accretion of cells, but rather the transformation, through time, of the developing being from one stage to the next to the next. If cells can be killed off in such wholesale quantities by genetic program at the beginning of life, there is no reason why this cannot continue to take place at a decelerated rate throughout life—with perhaps another spurt of acceleration toward the end of it.

Holger P. von Hahn of the Institute of Experimental Gerontology in Basel, Switzerland, proposes the existence of genes which specifically regulate aging. "In particular," he writes, in *Experimental Gerontology,* "the requirement for a highly precise time sequence in genetic regulation during embryogenesis and differentiation makes a large number of regulator genes in several super-imposed levels necessary.

"Embryogenesis and differentiation are clearly genetically controlled processes. One may therefore also postulate the existence of 'aging regulator genes,' which are switched on to replace the 'adult' regulator genes . . . at determined moments in the lifespan of the cell—for example, after the last 'scheduled' mitosis. Such 'aging regulator genes' might, for instance, produce a repressor which cannot be inactivated ('de-repressed') by the normal inducer molecules. . . . The result for the cell is a loss of genetic information due to the blocking of the transcription step of protein synthesis. This is exactly the type of situation we are proposing here for an aging cell."

The mechanics of all this will be better explained in a moment. But, in view of the observations of Whitten, Webb, von Hahn, and many others, it is not surprising that genetic on-off switching devices figure importantly in some theories of aging, including Strehler's. In the embryo and fetus, the switches are important not just for cell division and its cessation, but also so that each cell will know how to carry out its specific program as a skin cell, a muscle cell, or whatever specialized function is ordained for it.

In the adult organism, some cells go on dividing, and thus replacing themselves, throughout life. These are called *mitotic* cells (for *mitosis*—division). Others never divide again once the organism is fullgrown. These are called *postmitotic* (after mitosis is over) or "resting" cells. In between are other cells that do not ordinarily divide, but can begin doing so again when circumstances demand it. Liver cells serve as a good example of this in-between category. They appear to be postmitotic. But if a piece of the liver is cut away or damaged, the division switches are somehow turned on again in response to the challenge, and they spring into action until the missing piece is regenerated, then turn off again. (A salamander can regenerate a limb in this fashion, when it is lopped off. Some biologists believe it will one day be possible for human amputees to do likewise, once we know enough about on-off switching.)

Among the mitotic cells that divide throughout life are the outside or surface cells, such as skin cells and the epithelial cells that line the gastrointestinal tract. It may seem strange to hear the gut and stomach—which we usually think of as our innermost innards—referred to as being "outside." Yet, in a sense, they really are. The entire tract that has to do with eating, digesting, and eliminating runs all the way from the mouth to the anus in a single, unbroken space. It is a tube that changes shape as it goes, but still is a definable and visible entity, a continuous tunnel that opens to the outside world at both ends. Food gets into the body's *real* innards only by seeping through the tunnel's permeable walls. So the lining of this tract *is* like an outside surface, and its cells are in many ways similar to skin cells. At any rate, all these surface cells keep dying off and replacing themselves through continuing cell division. So do the blood cells—

red as well as white—and the lymphocytes, the cells of the body's immune system.

Among the postmitotic cells—those that never do divide again—are those of the muscles and nervous system. After a myocardial infarction (a heart attack), part of the heart muscle may be irreparably damaged—irreparably because these cells, unlike liver cells, are *not* switched on to regenerate themselves. A few researchers, among them Donald A. Fischman of the University of Chicago and Frederick H. Kasten of the Louisiana State University Medical School in New Orleans, are trying to "teach" heart cells how to do this in tissue culture; if they succeed, the hope is that heart cells in the living body can be taught to do the same. After a stroke, when brain cells are denied oxygen and therefore die, or when parts of the brain are damaged by any other means, this same incapacity to regenerate renders the damage permanent. In fact, under perfectly normal circumstances of aging, it has been estimated that as many as 100,000 brain cells a day die off after the age of thirty-five—hardly a negligible loss, even though the brain cells start off numbering in the billions. Brain-cell death, and especially the daily numbers involved, is a matter of some controversy; it has been seriously challenged, for instance, by Alex Comfort. But the major fact about postmitotic cells is that, once they die, they are gone forever.

Any theory of cellular aging must encompass both mitotic and postmitotic cells, as well as those in-between categories, in all their astonishing diversity of types. Many decry the idea that there could be a single genetic clock of aging located in the nucleus of each cell; if that were so, how could it account for the different ways in which these cells age and die? That raises no theoretical difficulty for me: If the same packet of DNA can program the cells to develop so differently, and to live such different existences, it can surely program them to age and die differently as well. It is, in fact, what one would expect.

Chapter IV

THE PROTEIN
ASSEMBLY LINES

The same objection is regularly raised in regard to hormonal theories of aging, which we will come to later: How can hormones released in the brain by the pituitary—where some feel the clock of aging is located—have such diverse results in so many kinds of individual cells? Again, one would expect that hormones *would* trigger a different set of reactions in cells differently programmed.

With all these differences in program, do cells have any activities they share in common? They do. Mainly, they make proteins. In fact, it can be said that when a typical cell (mature, though still young and healthy) is functioning according to program, its principal business is the manufacture of proteins (usually referred to in scientific papers as "protein synthesis"). Each cell makes many different kinds of protein—out of amino acids, which are broken down from the proteins we eat—and it makes them, by and large, for two purposes: to rebuild its own substance, and to export them for the needs of other cells. Endocrine cells, for example, make hormones—which are also proteins—for export to other cells. There are body cells, of course, which do not engage in the export trade. *All* cells, however, whether they continue to divide throughout life or whether they have stopped dividing for life, must keep on manufacturing protein to replace their own structural material in the constant breakdown and buildup we call metabolism. Food serves us here as both construction materials and fuel to run the cell's internal combustion engine. Like a car's engine, however, the cell's engine also requires oxygen, which is delivered regularly by the red blood cells.

We have already noted that every cell, with the specialized exception of the red blood cell, has a nucleus which serves as headquarters for the DNA. DNA has long since become a household monogram, and I have been using the term freely since the book's introduction. But it won't hurt to remind you once more that DNA is deoxyribonucleic acid, the master molecule of heredity, uniquely capable of replicating, of making exact copies of itself. It is what the chromosomes and genes are made of.

The other important nucleic acid is RNA, ribonucleic acid, quite similar to DNA in structure and coding. But, where DNA is a double-stranded helix, RNA is single-stranded and cannot make copies of itself. RNA—which comes in at least three or four varieties, as well as varieties within varieties (there are some sixty types of "transfer RNA" alone)—cannot make a useful move without explicit instructions from DNA.

RNA operates both within the nucleus and outside it—in the *cytoplasm,* which is the main body of the cell. Out in the cytoplasm are a number of different kinds of *organelles*—the generic name for cell parts which are neither in the nucleus nor part of the *cell membrane*. The nucleus and each organelle are surrounded by protective membranes of their own. The membrane is the cell wall, though in mammals this is not a solid wall as it is in most plants. It used to be thought of as simply the containing envelope that kept the cell's cytoplasm from spilling out into the general environs. But the membrane is now seen to be a very dynamic "wall" indeed, full of entrances and exits, mazes and secret passageways, guard towers, sentry boxes, and sets of signals and passwords by which strangers are admitted or kept out—all in all a highly complex and functional part of the cell. The specific nature of the membrane needn't concern us for the moment, nor need the cytoplasm, other than as the site of protein manufacture.

A cell, remember, is essentially a protein factory. All proteins are made of the same twenty amino acids broken down from food, though not all proteins contain all the amino acids. Among the more important kinds of proteins are *enzymes,* which come in thousands of varieties and serve as universal catalysts for all the cell's step-by-step chemical reactions. There is a different enzyme for each little step. This is what keeps our metabolic engine going at a slow-burning rate. Without enzymes we would heat up and go critical, like a nuclear reactor with the cadmium safety rods pulled out. If a vital enzyme is missing or inoperative—through some molecular error or genetic defect—an entire cellular chain reaction may come to a halt, or never begin.

The basic process of protein manufacture, oversimplified, is this: DNA orders and uses RNA to make proteins (out of amino acids) with the help of enzymes. That's the essential story. The genetic instructions are carried from the nucleus and executed in the cytoplasm, where the amino acids (very small molecules) are put together (on organelles called *ribosomes,* which serve as assembly workbenches) into the much larger protein molecules. DNA, RNA, and proteins (including enzymes) are all large molecules, with complicated three-dimensional configurations. When the assembly line is functioning efficiently, the cell is healthy; and there is no theoretical reason why, with luck, it could not go on functioning in this manner in perpetuity.

These large molecules are not only the intelligent supervisors but also the workers with the know-how to keep the protein assembly lines moving. If the director of the plant, DNA, never leaves its headquarters, it must transmit instructions accurately. It can only do so by chemical coding, permitting its executive director, RNA, to copy the master code from its (DNA's) own content, and entrusting it (RNA) to deliver the instructions intact. DNA's orders are spelled out in a simple four-letter code—though the combinations are complex. The same is true of RNA, though one of its code letters is different, thus making five code letters in all. It takes only three letters to designate a given amino acid.

The order of the letters is all-important, just as it is in any language. If we take the English letters O, D, and G, and place them in that order, ODG, the result is meaningless. We get a nonfunctional nonword. Rearrange the letters, however, into DOG, and they suddenly take on meaning. We evoke the image of a familiar, tail-wagging animal. Rearrange the letters yet again, and we come up with GOD, a radically different order of meaning. Using the same three letters, we have gone from no meaning at all to an animal to the deity. Some combinations (Z, L, M) are meaningless no matter how you arrange them, while others (A, R, T) tend to form meanings without much trouble. In biology, as in all science, the quantity of information—which includes its arrangement—dictates the quality of the result. Arrangement, or errors in arrangement, of the genetic letters in a cell can make the same drastic difference as errors in

English spelling. One misplaced genetic letter on the RNA chain can mean an error in one amino acid, therefore an error in the finished product. That product could be an enzyme which, if it failed to do its catalytic job at a critical step, might bring to a halt a whole sequence of activities. The further activities which depended on the completion of *that* sequence of activities could thus not begin to take place. The escalating effect could result in an "error catastrophe"— which is one of the major theories of aging, put forth by Leslie E. Orgel of the Salk Institute.

If the smooth functioning of the protein assembly line constitutes life, then interference with that functioning is what defines aging— the running out of life. How does it happen?

The important point to make here is not so much that an explicit genetic code exists, but that *we* are learning to "read and write" in it. We know that things do go wrong with the cell's protein factories. We are now maneuvering ourselves into a position where we can not only detect *when* something has gone wrong, but perhaps pinpoint specifically *what* has gone wrong, and begin to do something about it.

That is what molecular genetics is all about. It represents our major long-range hope for the cure and prevention of a variety of ailments, all the way from birth defects to cancer and the cardio-vascular diseases. In fact, so many of these late-in-life ailments, including cancer, heart disease, stroke, arthritis, diabetes, senile dementia, autoimmune disease, and a host of other degenerative diseases, are increasingly seen to have genetic components (though they are not simple, single-gene defects such as cystic fibrosis or sickle-cell anemia) and therefore might all be characterized, in a sense, as being birth defects. Aging research encompasses the whole molecular-genetic spectrum of research. The power to understand and manipulate the genetic information, a power growing by the day, will produce many ancillary payoffs, some now unforeseeable, before the aging process itself is finally elucidated.

Many current theories of aging are directly related to what can go wrong, and where, in the process of protein making. Some major theories focus on the genes, on the DNA: The original genetic instructions could be faulty. Or other genes may fail to function—such as those charged with repairing accidental breaks in the protein-making genes, or those responsible for switching the protein-making genes on or off at the appropriate times (a favorite idea of Strehler's). Errors could occur in copying the genetic information from DNA to RNA, or in transmitting the information—which of course means literally transporting it—out into the cytoplasm. Or at any step along the devious way to the assembly line, or at any point on that complex and precision-demanding assembly line itself.

Where the trouble occurs—and when—represents only one aspect of the problem. Trouble could occur, as time goes on, in all these places. The other aspect is *why* it occurs. Running contrapuntally through all theories of aging are a pair of controversial themes, either of which is in harmony with most of the observed facts. One holds that damage to the genetic machinery or errors in the protein-making process are the result of accident and incident, of wear and tear. The competing view, as we know, holds that most of the damage and errors expressed in the aging cell are dictated by the genes themselves, the on-off switches bringing *new* genes into play which start dismantling or disrupting the protein assembly lines so that the organism runs down by explicit program. In the latter case—with life and its demise all part of a single genetic package—if we could control the DNA, all the DNA, then we should be able to keep those assembly lines moving. Maybe not forever, but for an impressively long time.

Chapter V

THE CELL AS A MACHINE
THAT WEARS OUT

Among those who believe that gerontology has gone through its contradictory time-of-testing, and now is ready to move decisively ahead, is D. F. Chebotarev, director of the Soviet Union's Institute of Gerontology in Kiev. In fact, on the occasion of the Ninth International Congress of Gerontology, held in Kiev in 1972, Chebotarev expressed his firm conviction that gerontology "has now reached its concluding stage of accumulating practical material to be used for inferring profound theoretical generalizations."

We are, however, just at the beginning of this "concluding stage" and all the requisite "practical material" is not likely to be accumulated for some time to come. Hence the theoretical generalizations being propounded are seldom in agreement with one another. But no wonder. The visible signs of physiological aging, as well as the easily measurable running down of internal functions, are so many, and so varied—in fact, as another Soviet gerontologist, A. V. Nagorny, pointed out, each kind of tissue seems to have its own peculiar "handwriting of aging"—that a multiplicity of theories is to be expected. Nathan Shock, dean of American gerontologists and long-time director of NIH's Gerontological Research Center (GRC) in Baltimore, who was also a prominent figure at the Kiev Conference, believes that aging must be looked upon "as a complex phenomenon which may require different explanatory principles for different aspects of the process."

When one begins to look at aging theories, one must turn to the work of Alex Comfort who, in addition to being one of the world's leading gerontologists, has been in the business of collecting, analyzing, and expounding theories of aging longer than almost anyone around. Comfort has gained most of his recent fame—and fortune too—as an amateur sexologist, through his authorship of the best-selling *Joy of Sex* and *More Joy*. And he has recently transplanted himself from his native England to California. Those who know of him only in this incarnation may have been puzzled by two previous mentions of him in a book on aging research. But all of Comfort's professional credentials are in gerontology, and they were earned over most of the years of his life to date through his labors at the University of London. His technical output has been prodigious, and he has written numerous reviews and surveys of the field culminating in a highly regarded book (*Ageing: The Biology of Senescence,* published in 1964), as well as one of the best popular articles ever written on the subject.

The summer before he moved to California, I had lunch with Alex Comfort at his favorite Indian restaurant, near the University of London. Though he had no pet theory of his own, Comfort seemed, at that time, to be leaning—with Strehler and the others— toward the idea of genetically programmed aging. As we discussed one aging theory after another, he kept returning to a point that both amused and frustrated him: Many theorists, even those who do not believe in a genetic program, tend to select a single aspect of aging out of the diversity of possibilities as *the* primary cause of aging. "The hell of it is," said Comfort, "that you can seize upon almost any given feature of aging and invent a theory based on it. From one single aspect, it seems that you can usually derive most of the others!"

The other side of this, of course, is the argument that *no* theory of aging is necessary, inasmuch as senescence can easily be accounted for on the basis of accumulated accidents, errors, and wear and tear over time. The cell, after all, is a machine, so why should it not simply wear out, just as an automobile does? The whole body, for that matter, is a machine—though not a simple nuts-and-bolts kind of machine—and the same argument would be applicable for the same reasons.

But the way even a nonbiological machine wears out is not so simple as it might appear. Another British investigator and theorist, John Maynard Smith of the University of Sussex, in considering single-cause versus multiple-cause theories of aging, uses the automobile analogy to clarify some of the major problems: "As a car grows older," he writes, in *Proceedings of the Royal Society*, "the cylinders, the gearbox, the body work, the electrical wiring, all deteriorate. But the deterioration of each of these 'organs' is to a large extent independent of the others, as is shown by the fact that a gearbox from an old car, if put into a young one, would not be rejuvenated, and a gearbox from a young car put into an old one would not deteriorate any more rapidly. Thus ageing in motor cars is multiple in nature."

However, there is a large but: ". . . we can imagine circumstances," he goes on, "in which a single theory would be appropriate. Suppose that a new car was fed with petrol, oil, grease and water, but that the battery was never charged. It would soon show a number of symptoms of senescence, in the starter motor, the ignition, the lights, the traffic indicators. Yet these would all be symptoms of a single ageing process, and could all be cured by a single measure—changing the battery."

Later in the same discussion, Maynard Smith returns to the motor car analogy: "It may be true that different 'organs' age as a consequence of the same physical processes, even though ageing is 'multiple.' . . . In fact, only two, perhaps three, physical processes (abrasion, corrosion, and metal fatigue) are likely to be involved. Although the engine and gearbox age independently, both do so primarily because of mechanical wear, and the life of both might be extended by a single treatment—for example, an improved lubricant. Similarly, even if it proves that in animals different organs age independently, they may do so as a consequence of similar changes at a cellular level."

What kind of changes?

Alex Comfort, who is personally more attracted to the genetic clock idea because the *rate* of aging in organisms of the same species is so stable, has nevertheless speculated that aging in cells might be due to a kind of blurring of the genetic information over long periods of time. He has likened this process to what happens with repeated photocopying, where successive copies made from copies which are made from yet other copies will be of lower and lower quality. If a similar blurring or dimming effect occurred in cell division, then "the new cells produced by an old man would in some way be less viable than the new cells produced by him when he was a child." This effect, however, would only explain what happens in cells that continued to divide after maturity; and, as another gerontologist,

Benjamin Schloss, points out, "No one ever dies of dead skin." Comfort's Xerox analogy would thus not apply—and it is clear from his own recent papers that he agrees—to the senescence of the critical postmitotic cells, which are not required to undergo the hazards of continuing replication throughout life. Once these cells mature, copies never need to be made again. Thus the "blurring" phenomenon would certainly be ruled out as a principal aging mechanism in those creatures whose bodies are made entirely of nondividing cells. Maynard Smith offers the fruit fly as an example: "Since there is no cell division in adult *Drosophila,* mutations due to miscopying cannot occur."

Errors can and do occur, however, which have nothing to do with the DNA making copies of itself. Damage can be *inflicted* on DNA —or, for that matter, on any of the cell's large molecules—in many ways by sources outside the cell and as a by-product of the cell's own activities. Some of the damage is reparable, some not.

Our quick survey of the DNA-RNA-protein chain, sketchy as it was, makes it obvious that DNA damage would be a likely candidate for a theory of aging. DNA is the storehouse of genetic knowledge as well as the director of its applied uses. Moreover, a number of experiments over the years have suggested that the progressive breakdown of genetic material with aging is more than theoretical. As one example, Tracy M. Sonneborn and his associates at Indiana University, studying the reproductive capacities of paramecia during the 1950's, found that the older the parents, the smaller was the percentage of vigorous offspring they could produce. Any injury to the DNA molecule, especially to those segments of it that dictate protein synthesis, could have serious consequences for the welfare of the cell—unless, of course, the cell was finished forever with that particular piece of information. An example cited by the late Howard J. Curtis of the Brookhaven National Laboratory: "If the gene for eye color is mutated in a liver cell, nothing of consequence will result."

We know that changes—mutations—do occur in DNA. They may be caused by many factors not in the original genetic program: viruses, potent chemicals, extreme heat, radiation (cosmic or manmade). Mutations can be good or bad—"good" or "bad" being variously defined under varying circumstances—and the outcome of evolution for a given species may depend on how these balance out. To influence evolution, mutations must occur in the germ cells—

sperm or egg—in which case they are *genetic* mutations, capable of being passed on to the ensuing generations. A mutation in other body cells is called a *somatic* mutation, which affects only that one already-existing person; this is the type believed to be implicated in individual human aging.

Anyone may, in the course of his lifetime, accumulate mutations in cells anywhere in the body. The late Leo Szilard, when he turned his ingenious mathematical-physicist's mind to biology in 1959, theorized that chance mutations in the genetic material, perhaps caused by the random impact of cosmic rays tearing through the cells' nuclei over a lifetime, could gradually damage—or even kill outright—one cell after another until the organism began to run down and finally not enough viable cells were left to sustain it. Szilard's theory applied specifically to nondividing cells. Inasmuch as Szilard's calculations would have resulted in a roughly identical life span for most people, he further theorized that variations in life span were largely due to the fact that people started out in life with differing quantities of already inherited DNA faults. "However," argued biochemist M. S. Kanungo, of India's Banaras Hindu University, "this theory does not explain why identical twins do not die within a year of each other." Other criticism has since pretty well invalidated Szilard's theory; but it served as a valuable stimulus for aging theory at the time.

Soviet gerontologists have also intensively investigated what happens to DNA with age. In summarizing these results in 1972, Kharkov University's V. N. Nikitin concluded that "using the present methods of extracting and analysing native DNA samples, no unambiguous and clear answer has been received to the question of the age dependence of DNA molecules and the 'residual proteins' associated with them."

Nevertheless, a damaged, blurred, misshapen, or somehow weakened DNA molecule—or many of them, in cases of gross chromosomal damage—is central to the somatic mutation theory of aging, which was most carefully worked out before his death by Brookhaven's Howard Curtis, a close observer of chromosomal damage caused by radiation. With its DNA unable to convey accurate instructions, the cell's protein factory might muddle through, erratically turning out products of uncertain quality, or it might just shut down. "Indeed," Curtis felt, in 1966, "from what we now know, it appears that the only way in which a permanent change, short of death, can be effected in the cell is by a change in the DNA or chromosome structure. All other damage can be repaired."

But it turns out that all other damage can *not* necessarily be repaired, and that there *are* other ways short of mutation and death by which the cell can be permanently changed. Most gerontologists today feel that the somatic mutation theory does not really stand up to close critical scrutiny. One argument is that, in postmitotic cells such as those of the brain and muscles, most of the genetic material is switched off anyway, since the cell never needs the information again (as in Curtis's own example of the liver cell and eye color); so random damage to most of the DNA would have no effect on protein manufacturing, thus none on the aging process either. Strehler, basing his critique on work done by A. G. Sacher at Oak Ridge as well as in his own laboratory, is among those who have discarded the somatic mutation theory. Maynard Smith, using mathematical reasoning—which gave the theory its original power—has pretty well demolished it, in Comfort's view.

Moreover, a number of recent experiments and calculations have convinced many that mutations occur much less frequently than was formerly assumed. And of the mutations that do occur, most are probably not permanent; we have known at least since 1960, thanks to Ruth Hill's work at Columbia University, that DNA creates its own self-repair enzymes. These enzymes would be manufactured, like any other protein on the assembly line, on instruction from the "repair genes." They probably correct most mutational damage before the faulty information can be transmitted. It is true that the cell's repair capacity can be virtually knocked out by a single massive dose of radiation. Yet it is not significantly diminished if the same quantity of radiation is administered in smaller doses over a period of time. Normal wear and tear would be most unlikely, at any point in life, to include a traumatic event of such severity and suddenness as to inactivate all the repair genes at once.

Paradoxically, this very repair capacity is what makes investigators such as Boston University's F. Marott Sinex reluctant to give up the somatic mutation theory altogether. He is intrigued by the fact that only a relatively few genes—perhaps four in all—seem to control the entire mechanism of DNA repair. In that case it would not require a large number of unlucky "hits" (as Szilard called them) to impair the function of these crucial genes. Thus information loss in aging would be due not so much to the extent of DNA damage as to its loss of ability to repair the damage.

It makes good evolutionary sense, of course, to suspect that all cells are not equal in their self-repair capabilities. Cells of the skin, gut, and bone marrow—which continually replace themselves by division—would seldom last long enough to undergo the kind of steady wear and tear that results in dangerous accumulations of damage. Hence they would have little need to require an always-at-the-ready fix-and-patch team. The highly specialized cells, however, which are assigned many important duties and must try to last as long as the organism does, because they no longer reproduce, are in a quite different situation. Their long-term repair needs are great, and it stands to reason that evolutionary experience would have taken due note of it.

Zhores A. Medvedev, the brilliant and courageous Soviet gerontologist who has been working in England for the past few years at London's National Institute for Medical Research, considers DNA damage from another standpoint: At any given time, most of the DNA in the cell's nucleus is unused. Much of it is in fact redundant—never used at all, at least not in protein manufacture. Samuel Boyer III of Johns Hopkins University now believes that this "junk DNA," as it has been called, may represent the critical evolutionary information that dictates whether the creature possessing it will turn out to be a mouse, a monkey, or a man. In any case, there also seem to be redundant, reiterative DNA sequences for the protein-making genes—so that one could take over if the other were damaged; though not all genes are repeated with the same frequency, and some may not be repeated at all.

It would be as if, in a football game, some players had many substitutes on the bench, while others had few or none. If a team had only one expert punter and place-kicker, and he suffered injury, it would simply have to do its best without the services of a kicker. If, as the game went on, other players were injured—and their substitutes as well—the team would play under increasing handicaps, until finally, perhaps without a center or quarterback, the game would be lost by default. Medvedev has suggested that those genes without substitute sequences would be the most vulnerable. If such a gene were damaged, and if the information thus irretrievably lost contained an indispensable piece of the protein recipe (to switch metaphors), then the protein factory would, to that extent, be handicapped.

Bernard Strehler too believes that the repetitive sequences of DNA may be important in aging. He had set out in 1972, with one of his students, Roger Johnson, to disprove the somatic mutation theory. But he "did not rule out another possible type of damage, the gradual loss of copies of certain genes that exist by the hundreds, side by side in each cell's DNA. Although the idea seemed improbable to us," he recalls, in the 1973 edition of *Science Year, The World Book of Science Annual,* "we set out to test it by comparing the number of copies of one such gene in brain cells from young and old beagles. The repetitive gene that we chose produces a major constituent of ribosomes, ribosomal RNA (rRNA)." Strehler and Johnson found that "the brain cells of old dogs contained about 30 per cent fewer copies of the gene than did those of the young dogs. We also measured the number of copies of the gene in other tissues of these animals, and found that all of those tissues whose cells had stopped reproducing (brain, heart, skeletal muscle) showed similar decreases. However, none of the tissues whose cells were still reproducing (liver, kidney) showed a decrease.

"In other words, the protein-making machinery of heart cells, brain cells, muscle cells, hormone-producing cells, sex cells, cells that produce antibodies, and all other nonreproducing cells may stop working effectively for the same reason—too few ribosomes. (Ribosomes, remember, are the cytoplasm's assembly-line workbenches.) If further studies should establish this as a universal accompaniment of aging in higher animals, extending the healthy life span might be achieved by increasing the number of ribosomes available in the cells of critical tissues."

In Strehler's scheme of things, the DNA molecules (which originally dictate the manufacture of the cell's ribosomes) are not damaged or destroyed, but merely switched off by inhibiting substances so that the information needed to make the RNAs and proteins is no longer available. Holger von Hahn's findings in Switzerland, and his interpretation of them, seem to bear out Strehler's thesis. Von Hahn found that the DNA double helix is much more stable—i.e., harder to break apart—in aging cells, and he decided that this stability was "dependent on the presence and the binding of certain proteins. It appears that in old nucleoprotein a particular protein fraction is bound to DNA in such a way as to increase the energy required for the separation of the two strands in the helix. Since strand separation is a necessary step in the mechanism of transcription, blocking this process necessarily blocks transcription, and thus leads to a loss of genetic information for the cell."

Strehler hypothesizes that the cell is programmed, at a certain point in life, to start manufacturing the very substances which then proceed to switch off the critical genes. The "damage" is thus not random or accidental, but rather the purposeful carrying out of the genetic program. Some plants and insects are definitely known to possess "mutator" genes which are programmed to produce mutations in their own DNA, but such genes have so far not been found in human chromosomes. If Strehler's view is correct, it is a much more hopeful one, since the genes are still present, though covered up. It is, then, only necessary to *un*cover them—perhaps by unbinding von Hahn's proteins—and thus switch the genes on again to function as efficiently as in their "youth."

Even if all the DNA in the cell were to remain perfectly intact throughout life, however, information loss could still occur elsewhere —and the results would be the same as if the DNA itself were deficient. There are, as we have already seen, other molecules which DNA relies on to carry the protein-making instructions out into the assembly lines. These are the several varieties of RNA, and certain enzymes—especially those required to make more RNA, or to help RNA make more proteins (including more enzymes). These molecules are charged with transcribing and translating the genetic instructions. As long as they remain in efficient working order, they can readily repair damage to *other* molecules. But damage to one of these key molecules would be irreparable. It would be like knocking out someone on the assembly line—or en route to it—who was the only one who knew how to do that particular job. If he were crippled, or absent, components would come off the line improperly assembled, or production might come to a confused halt as everything jammed at a given point.

You may already have recognized this as another way of describing what was earlier referred to as the "error catastrophe theory" of the Salk Institute's Leslie Orgel. Orgel—like Comfort, an Englishman self-transplanted to California—has also made major contributions to theories about the origins of life on earth. Though Orgel now believes there may be mechanisms at work that could prevent error catastrophes from occurring—and is the first to say that the newest experimental evidence is inconclusive and often confusing—his hypothesis, even more than Szilard's, has served a powerful enzymatic function of its own in aging theory. Hardly a review article on aging research in any technical journal fails to take Orgel's theory into serious account—a statement that cannot be made for many aging theories. Moreover, it has stimulated an enormous quantity of fruitful research. At the National Institute of Medical Research at Mill Hill, London (where Medvedev also works), Robin Holliday, in collaboration with C. M. Lewis and G. M. Tarrant, has carried out a series of experiments with cells in culture. Their results seem to corroborate Orgel's error theory, as do similar studies carried out by B. I. Goldstein in the U.S.S.R.

Nevertheless, Holliday and his associates believe (as Orgel now agrees) that—in Orgel's words—"it may not be possible to separate the contributions to cellular ageing caused by errors of protein synthesis from those due to the accumulation of somatic mutations. Errors of protein synthesis must occasionally lead to the formation of 'mutator' DNA polymerase molecules which replicates DNA inaccurately. Conversely, some mutations . . . must reduce the fidelity of protein synthesis. Thus inaccurate protein synthesis and inaccurate DNA synthesis are coupled phenomena."

The same dual interpretation can be applied to many other experiments—for example, the findings of Harriet and David Gershon at the Technion-Israel Institute of Technology in Haifa. The Gershons' studies of mice and nematodes showed a consistent "accumulation with age of altered, partially active, or catalytically inactive enzyme molecules"—results that would fit either the error theory or the mutation theory. There were some suggestions, at the end of 1969, that many proteins might be one-shot creations, that is, made to last for the lifetime of the cell. This was based on some fascinating experiments at Sussex by Maynard Smith and his associates A. N. Bozcuk and Susan Tebbutt, which showed that, in the fruit fly *Drosophila,* just as there were cells which never divided again, so there were large quantities of protein (the structural protein of the thoracic flight muscles, for instance) that did not turn over—i.e., were not broken down and resynthesized. In that case, neither error catastrophes occurring in, say, RNA, nor mutations in the DNA would cause aging, but only damage to—or the ultimate wearing out of—the irreplaceable protein itself.

But *Drosophila* is different from vertebrates in many respects—one, already mentioned, being that the body of the adult is made entirely of nondividing cells. Maynard Smith still believes that the one-time-only protein deterioration "provides a sufficient cause of aging in *Drosophila*," but adds that: "Unfortunately the wearing out of non-replaced protein structures is unlikely to be the major cause of aging in vertebrates."

The one universal element in all observations and theories about aging is that something goes wrong, somewhere along the line, with components of the DNA-RNA-enzyme-protein assembly line. Attempts to replace damaged or error-ridden cellular components, whether in the nucleus or elsewhere, have provided the basis for a number of implausible rejuvenation therapies. The celebrated Swiss "cell therapist," Paul Niehans, for example, injected fresh sheep-embryo cells into his aging patients—many of them rich and famous. Benjamin Frank, a New York physician, claims success with diets that provide everything that failing cells might need—nucleic acids, enzymes, and proteins—packaged into a single daily meal. Critics object that, inasmuch as food is all broken down in the liver anyway, and reaches the cell as raw materials, efficient cell machinery is still required to put it all together again.

Here again Strehler's outlook may be the most hopeful. If his surmise is correct, it may well be possible to "awaken the sleeping genes" so that they would be as good as new, capable of correcting any kind of errors, wherever they might occur, however catastrophic they might be adjudged in today's cellular circumstances. In this context, it is worth describing briefly an earlier experiment of Strehler's, this time with his student Michael Bick (who has since moved on, first to Harvard, then to the Roche Institute of Molecular Biology). They worked with the cotyledons (first leaves) of the soybean plant, a convenient experimental tool because the cotyledon has a life span of just three weeks from the day the seed sprouts to the day of the leaf's withering and death (falling off the plant). Strehler and Bick found that transfer RNA (tRNA) molecules had no trouble binding with the amino acids leucine and tyrosine at the age of seven days. But by the age of twenty-one days, they had a great deal of trouble doing so. Even more interesting, the older cotyledons contained *new* substances not present in the younger ones—substances which *inhibited and inactivated the enzymes* that normally attach the amino acids to the tRNA molecules. Strehler took this as clear evidence of a specific genetic aging program: genes had been turned on to create the enzyme-inactivating substances at the right time (or perhaps the wrong time, from the leaf's viewpoint). Strehler's answer, again: control of the on-off switching mechanisms.

Kanungo and his colleagues in India have put forth a similar theory featuring genetic on-off switching as both a probable cause and possible cure for aging. Orgel, too, gives cautious support to the genetic clock theory, but warns, in *Nature*, that "it seems unwise, in the absence of experimental evidence, to take for granted the idea of 'programmed obsolescence' in man and other mammals."

Just as Orgel sees the interrelationship of DNA errors and protein-making errors, and the feedback between them, so does he emphasize the mutual impact of these errors with other kinds of damage in the cell's cytoplasm and membrane—and, for that matter, with the aging of the body's noncellular material. An increasing number of gerontologists are in agreement. Virtually every aspect of aging seems to exaggerate and accelerate the other aspects. Hence Comfort's complaint that you can use almost any facet of aging to explain all the others.

As a case in point, on the same day I had read a paper of Comfort's in which he reiterated the wry comment I heard from him in London, I picked up a copy of *Science* in which William Bondareff and Robert Narotzky of the Northwestern University Medical School in Chicago report some careful experiments with rat brain cells. They were, in this instance, concentrating on measuring the *spaces* between cells. It turns out that the space between senescent brain cells is, on the average, only half that between the cells of younger adults. Starting with this information alone, I tried playing Comfort's game: What functions do these spaces serve? Because the brain contains essentially no connective tissue, the spaces are probably critical in the transport of all sorts of chemicals as well as in all-important communications among the neurons. (This chemical transport *is* known to be reduced with age.) With shrinking space between the cells, they obviously cannot function as well— and the resulting increase in pressure and density must also change the cell's physical configuration and produce adverse effects in its molecular activities, including protein manufacture. We know that the welfare of all the body's cells and tissues is dependent upon the control functions of the brain. If those decline, then all physiological functions begin to deteriorate. Ergo, the cause of aging is the shrinkage of spaces between brain cells.

Bondareff and Narotzky did not offer this as a theory of aging, but they might have.

Chapter VI

GARBAGE GLUT, FREE RADICAL RAPE, AND THE SELF-TURNED-ENEMY

Some investigators have attached great importance to the cell's difficulty, as the years go by, in getting rid of its wastes. In many cells, especially those that no longer divide, there is a steady buildup of cellular garbage, especially a pigmented fatty substance called *lipofuscin,* discovered independently in a number of laboratories, including Strehler's, around 1958. Most gerontologists feel that lipofuscin is a result rather than a cause of aging and that its deleterious effects are more theoretical than proven. But in many cells, lipofuscin accumulates to a point where it occupies 10, 20, or even 30 per cent of the space, and one can see how the cell might choke on its own pollutants. It would be as if, on an increasingly crowded dance floor, the mere taking up of the physical space made it harder and harder for anyone with purposeful activities (say, waiters carrying food or drinks) to get through. The role of lipofuscin as a specific cause of aging, however, is rendered further ambiguous (as the Dutch gerontologist C. F. Hollander points out) by the fact that its granules sometimes show up even in the cells of newborn infants. Here again, though lipofuscin is generally regarded as a wear-and-tear product, Strehler puts much of the blame for these garbage deposits on the cell's genetic program. In support of this contention, he cites the child victims of Batten's disease (a genetic disorder) who accumulate vast quantities of lipofuscin in their brain cells, are blind by the age of five, and undergo steady mental deterioration until their premature deaths.

Lipofuscin accumulation is attributed by some to the effects of "cross-linkage." In fact, one of the most durable single-cause theories of aging is the cross-linkage theory, originally proposed in the early 1940's by Johan Bjorksten, now director of the Bjorksten Research Foundation in Madison, Wisconsin. Cross-linkage is the inadvertent coupling of any two large molecules, inside or outside the cell. When a pair of adjacent molecules are cross-linked at some point, the cell's enzymes can often break them apart again. But irreversible cross-linkages occur more frequently with age. They occur in proteins, enzymes, RNA, even in DNA, so they could be the cause of both somatic mutations and error catastrophes.

If someone were to throw a lasso over two adjacent workers on an assembly line, and if they couldn't get the lasso off, they might not be totally immobilized, but they certainly could not be expected to do their assigned job. And they would take up more and more space, and be more and more troublesome to get around. In the cell, lots of cross-linkages mean lots of work stoppages—and, finally, no work at all. A few gerontologists—Robert Kohn is one—believe that the cross-linking of molecules outside the cell and the consequent stiffening of connective tissue alone could account for many of the functional losses of old age. A. A. Bogomolets, one of the founders of Soviet gerontology, attached similar importance to the aging of connective tissue.

At least two other scientists independently suggested the cross-linkage theory of aging: Frederic Verzar, a Hungarian who did most of his work in Switzerland (some of it with von Hahn); and Major Donald G. Carpenter of the United States Air Force Academy in Colorado Springs. But Bjorksten—who first got the idea when, as a young chemist for Ditto, Inc., he noticed a strange similarity between the "aging" of hectograph duplication film and the aging of human tissue—has clear priority. For more than thirty years now, Bjorksten has done painstaking research and continued to elaborate his theory with great force, conviction, and documentation. In a summarizing article published in 1971, he stated confidently: "The crosslinkage theory stands unique among the primary theories of aging. It stands simply and without strained assumptions." It is, he insists, compatible with all other theories of aging. He announced that no more work would be done to validate a theory already substantially proven, and that henceforth he would devote his efforts to finding and testing anti-cross-linking substances—a program which has already met with some modest success.

In *Extended Youth,* a book published in 1968, Robert W. Prehoda introduced his chapter on cross-linkage with this glowing tribute to Bjorksten: "A theory very likely to be of equal importance to biology as were Albert Einstein's contributions to physics was first refined at the start of World War II by a brilliant chemist, Dr. Johan Bjorksten. Future history books will describe the years of debate, slow acceptance, and the dramatic breakthrough that was the beginning of a true understanding of the aging process." But one can't remind oneself too often of Comfort's warning about the ease of parlaying a set of observations into a comprehensive theory of aging. In those few years since Prehoda's book, the cross-linkage theory has lost much ground—which is not to say that it couldn't regain it in such a mercurial field of endeavor. Today it is possible to read major surveys of gerontological research and theory with no mention of Bjorksten at all—a premature dismissal, surely. No one denies that cross-linkage occurs or that it increases with age, but most gerontologists now seem to agree with the judgment of Charles G. Kemendy of the Bristol Laboratories in Syracuse, New York, that cross-linkage "is not a cause but simply a result of aging."

A significant portion of cross-linkage is undoubtedly caused by "free radicals." In fact, there has developed a well-worked-out free radical theory of aging. Its principal originator and proponent is Denham Harman, of the University of Nebraska School of Medicine in Omaha. Harman—like Strehler and Comfort, a dedicated investigator as well as an evangelist for gerontology—was the founding father, and still remains the center of organizing energy, of the American Aging Association (AGE). While the cross-linkage theory has declined in influence (for now, anyway), the free radical theory has picked up an increasing number of advocates, including Aloys L. Tappel of the University of California at Davis, Lester Packer of the University of California at Berkeley, Paul Gordon of Northwestern, and Richard A. Passwater of the American Instrument Company in Silver Spring, Maryland.

Free radicals are highly unstable atoms, broken-off pieces of molecules, or molecules with an electron stripped away. Because a free electron can hardly stand being unattached, free radicals tend to race frantically around the cell until they find other molecules they can latch on to. "A free radical," says Alex Comfort, "has been likened to a convention delegate away from his wife: it's a highly reactive chemical agent that will combine with anything that's around." In some cases a free radical might more accurately be likened to a rapist. Its union with another molecule—ready or not (some molecules are more vulnerable than others, depending on their momentary state of activity)—often amounts to an outright attack. Though the lifetime of a free radical is measured in thousandths of a second, that is plenty of time to do considerable damage. To make matters worse, a free radical's attack on another molecule may sometimes be so violent as to create other free radicals, thus setting off a small chain reaction of devastation in the neighborhood.

Free radicals can split molecules in half, knock pieces out of them, contribute considerably to the buildup of lipofuscin, and garble the cellular information in a number of ways—only one of which is cross-linkage. Especially vulnerable are the delicate cell-surface membranes, as well as the membranes of the organelles within the cytoplasm, particularly the cell's all-important energy machines, the mitochondria. "One quality that characterizes free radical action," Paul Gordon notes, "is that . . . free radicals do not appear to contain or reflect any useful biological information. Their action on membranes, therefore, represents the replacement of genetically determined order by randomness."

In the course of studying radiation damage in the 1950's, Denham Harman noticed that: (1) radiation not only causes symptoms that look like mature aging in animals, but actually seems to shorten the life span; and (2) radiation creates an excess quantity of free radicals in cells. He wondered if the free radicals could be causing the aging effects. All cells produce small quantities of free radicals *in the normal course of their everyday oxidation reactions.* If a lot of free radicals created in one quick moment can cause accelerated aging, could a smaller quantity, spread over a long period of time, cause normal aging?

Harman knew that, in various industrial processes, antioxidant substances were used to combat free radical damage—to prevent the deterioration of leather, rubber, and synthetics, for instance, and to keep butter from turning rancid. (T. L. Dormandy of London's Whittington Hospital has referred to free radical cell damage as "biological rancidification.") At the beginning of his investigation, Harman was mainly concerned with minimizing or treating radiation damage, which he was able to do by administering antioxidants such as 2-MEA (2-mercaptoethylamine), BHT (butylated hydroxytoluene), Vitamin E, and a quinoline derivative called Santoquin; all are compounds that hold down oxidation reactions and mop up free radicals. When he became interested in the aging problem, Harman set up experiments with normal, unirradiated mice, and found that by mixing antioxidants into their food, he was able to keep them alive significantly longer than mice who did not get antioxidants. For a while, he thought he had succeeded in extending the life spans of these mice, but finally concluded that he had merely stretched out their life *expectancy,* enabling them to come much closer to the end of their potential maximum life spans—still a considerable accomplishment.

There may be high irony in one aspect of free radical research: It turns out that a high intake of polyunsaturated fats increases the cell's oxidation reactions, thus creating more free radicals and thus, presumably, more of all types of aging damage. The irony lies in the fact that, because of the implication of cholesterol in atherosclerosis and heart disease, millions of Americans—and now millions in other nations—have switched from saturated fats to polyunsaturated fats. We have done so in order to increase our life expectancy by avoiding premature heart attacks. But, in doing so, have we contributed instead to the premature aging of all our cells? This consideration, anything but trivial, is what has led researchers in this field —notably A. L. Tappel—to recommend the inclusion of Vitamin E in the daily diet, though exact experimental data as to dosage and efficacy are still lacking.

The study of free radicals in aging has revealed their potential importance in other medical areas as well—cancer, as one example. Inasmuch as free radicals inflict damage to the molecular genetic apparatus, the disruption of which can mark the beginning of a cell's transformation to an abnormal state, it makes sense that the individual whose cells undergo this kind of damage runs a higher risk of developing a runaway malignant growth. Richard Passwater, in particular, has followed up this ominous possibility.

Another critical system which can undergo free radical damage is the immune system. But, then, the lymphocytes of the immune system are also subject to all the same hazards as are the body's other cells.

This consideration brings us to another highly developed and very well thought of theory of aging—the autoimmune hypothesis. Among its supporters and originators are Sir Macfarlane Burnet of Australia and Takashi Makinodan of NIH. But its principal theorist, investigator, and elucidator has been Roy L. Walford, a UCLA pathologist. The immune theory has been spelled out most convincingly by Walford in a book, *The Immunologic Theory of Aging,* published in 1969, updated and somewhat modified in his more recent papers.

We know that, as we age, our immunological defenses diminish, and the incidence of autoimmune disease rises. This could mean: (1) that the immune cells themselves change through damage, error, or information loss of one kind or another in such a way that their powers of recognition fail them, and they can't distinguish between friend and foe—i.e., between "self" and "not-self"; or (2) that other cells of the body change for the same reasons to such an extent that they begin to "look foreign" to the immune cells and are thus attacked; or (3) both. The immunological theory will also be discussed in another context in a later chapter.

The theories of aging are far from exhausted by this catalog. A number remain undescribed, and a few unmentioned. But there is no need to be all-inclusive. The point is already sufficiently made that many viable theories of aging have now been worked out to a degree where they can be tested, and either proved or disproved. Comfort believes that the free radical theory, for one, can be disposed of one way or the other by a sizable short-term effort. That done, we could either drop it as a primary cause of aging (though it still might be a contributory cause) or else concentrate on it with fresh vigor.

It is clear, too, that these theories spell out many possible causes of aging which do not require a genetically programmed clock of aging. All these taken together—free radicals, cross-linkages, somatic mutations, error catastrophes, lipofuscin accumulation, autoimmune reactions, the stiffening of connective tissue, all the varieties of simple wear and tear—seem more than sufficient to account for the process of aging. In point of fact, any single one of these "causes," even if none of the others existed, could all by itself eventually result in the death of the organism.

Eventually, yes. But on schedule? If any one of these factors, or all of them taken together, told the whole aging story, wouldn't we expect to see much greater variations in the life span of a given species? Why doesn't a shrew, just an occasional shrew, live to be 150 or 200 years old, like the Galapagos tortoise? And why shouldn't a Galapagos tortoise, every now and then, wear out at the age of one and a half, as the shrew does?

And why—asks W. Donner Denckla of the Roche Institute of Molecular Biology in Nutley, New Jersey, whose work we shall soon come to—should some classes of animals die sooner than others with a higher metabolic rate, perhaps the surest measure of wear and tear?

And why—asks Leonard Hayflick of Stanford, another key figure—are cancer cells immortal in tissue culture and normal cells not, though both are subjected to exactly the same conditions of wear and tear? Hayflick's own experiments with aging cells in culture have led him to the belief that "the fundamental events which orchestrate age-related changes are likely to be found in the genetic machinery." We now arrive at these experiments of Hayflick's, which are among the most important, the most fascinating, and the most controversial in all of recent gerontology.

Chapter VII

HAYFLICK AND THE CELLULAR AGING CLOCK

Starting a biological revolution was not what Ross Harrison of Johns Hopkins had in mind when he first hit upon the idea, back in 1907, of trying to keep alive a fragment of frog-nerve tissue by immersing it in the frog's own juices. He merely wanted to find out whether or not nerve fibers grew from single cells. The question was in dispute. Harrison's experiment succeeded, and he did demonstrate that nerve fibers grew from single cells. As an incidental by-product of the experiment, he also proved—and herein lies the revolution— that tissue could be kept alive outside the body of the host organism. In this situation, the cells take their nourishment from the surrounding medium—whether it is natural (supplied by the body fluids of the host) or artificially concocted (nearly always the case in current experimentation)—and continue to proliferate in the best of health. If they are *not* in the best of health, speaking purely from the donor's point of view (e.g., cancer cells), they proliferate even more readily.

This past quarter of a century has been an extraordinarily creative period in biology—and tissue culture, once its uses were understood, has been one of the most powerful tools for the acquisition of knowledge about living cells in an enormous variety of species. Human cells have of course been of special interest to biomedically oriented researchers.

The longest continuously maintained human cell strain in biology is the HeLa strain, begun by George O. Gey—also of Johns Hopkins—in 1951, and still thriving in laboratories all over the world. Gey took the first samples from a patient who had cancer of

50

the cervix. (He and La were the first two letters of her first and last names—Henrietta Lacks, frequently misreported as Helen Lane.) Because the HeLa strain has proven to be unusually stable and extremely valuable for many specialized studies, the cancer cells of Henrietta Lacks are still undergoing nonstop multiplication twenty-five years after her death. They have undoubtedly divided and re-divided to create many times the 60 trillion or so cells that originally made up her entire adult body. Cancer cells cannot possess this kind of virtual immortality as inhabitants of a living body. Their uncon-trolled growth, in fact, constitutes an act of suicide, since it kills the organism on which they depend for their life-support systems—much as the human species seems intent on doing with the planet earth. In tissue culture, the cancer cells, released from their bodily boun-daries and supplied with an abundance of all their growth needs, can go on indefinitely.

Only mitotic cells, those that continue to divide in the living body, will continue to divide in culture as well. Postmitotic cells, such as mature brain and heart cells, do not begin dividing again on being transferred to culture; they remain in their "resting" state. Some attempts are being made, as already noted, to impart to them this capacity—to teach them to start dividing again, perhaps by reactivat-ing turned-off genetic switches. This is, after all, what cancer cells are good at doing, though in transferring their own proliferative capacities to neighboring cells, they render their neighbors abnormal as well.

Scientists have long suspected that the neoplastic (cancerous) transformation is brought about by altering the genetic on-off switches of the afflicted cell; the STOP DIVIDING signal, which was supposed to be posted forever, somehow gets taken down (de-repressed). This suspicion has lately been magnified by the discovery that a number of enzymes and hormones which are normally present only in the fetus reappear again in adults who have cancer. In fact, the presence of these fetal chemicals may emerge as excellent "markers" for the early diagnosis of certain types of cancer. O. W. Jones and his colleagues at the University of California at San Diego, for instance, have found that a certain form of the enzyme thymidine kinase (TK), which otherwise appears only in prenatal life, also shows up in adult cancer tissue. Carcinoembryonic antigen (CEA) reappears apparently only in the victims of cancer of the gastrointestinal tract. Alpha-fetoprotein (AFP) is most likely to be found in liver cancer patients. AFP also turns up consistently in the rare immunological birth defect known as ataxia-telangiectasia, whose victims have a very high predisposition to cancer. In their case, it is as though nature had forgotten to switch off the gene for AFP at the scheduled time. "That 'forgetfulness,' " as Joe Mori of the National Foundation–March of Dimes observes, "may be part of the hereditary defect. Such 'recall' of embryonic traits," he further speculates, "may be a feature of other diseases of adults as well." In the cancer cases, it seems logical that the TK, CEA, and APF found in adults are the results of genes that had been switched off at the appropriate time in fetal development, presumably forever, but had now been switched on again through some fault or accident in adult life—either "caused" by the cancer, or itself acting as a contributory cause of the cell's neoplastic transformation.

The good news side of this bad news is that Strehler may well be on the right track in his aging theories. If "permanently" switched-off genes can be reactivated to our disadvantage by cancer mechanisms, then we can learn to de-repress others to our advantage—the desirable genes that will keep our vital cellular protein factories going full blast. So far, those researchers who have had some limited success in inducing postmitotic cells to divide again in tissue culture have done so only at the expense of transforming them to an abnormal state. But this kind of effort is only in its infancy, and there is every reason to feel confident that we will acquire the sophistication to turn on the "start" switches again while leaving the cell otherwise intact—and also to activate the "stop" switches when we know (or the organism knows) it is time for cell division to come to a halt once more. Something like this happens in wound healing. Cells multiply to repair the injury, then stop multiplying when the job is done. Because the repair mechanism is imprecise, some scar tissue remains. It would obviously be desirable to bestow the gift of self-repair upon the living heart. (Whether it would be an equivalent blessing for the brain is less certain, as we shall presently see.)

The fact that cells that no longer divide in the body will not divide in culture suggests that there must be some relationship between what happens in culture (*in vitro*) and what happens in the living organism (*in vivo*), in which case studies in the one state, convenient and accessible, will tell us something about the other, which is both complex and often out of experimental reach. How close is the relationship? That is a matter of continuing debate. Cells could not, of course, be expected to undergo the same experiences in such contrasting environments. Cells in culture are living outside their normal context. They get no feedback from the other cells and organs that would ordinarily surround them. They are out of touch with the body's hormonal and nervous systems. They are sustained on artificial nutrients. For these and other good reasons, it would be surprising if their behavior and development did not differ in many respects from what they would be in the cells' natural habitat. Nevertheless, as a means of observing the workings of living cells and manipulating them at the whim of the investigator, tissue culture is unbeatable. Besides, no bioethical questions arise when experimenting with cell clones. (*Cloning* is a term much used these days. A *clone* is any growth of cells, usually from a single starter cell, that has come about asexually. The cloning so widely discussed has to do with the prospective capacity to grow whole organs—or even whole organisms—from single adult cells.)

A test tube full of cultured cells is not only cheaper, easier to handle, and more accessible to observation than an animal subject would be; there are many experiments that simply could not be carried out in any other way. How else could we watch viruses infect cells, observe how cells resist them and how they succumb to them, discover how normal cells may be transformed into tumor cells? Much of our newest cancer knowledge derives directly from tissue-culture studies. One can also use culture to *grow* viruses—as was done in developing the polio vaccine.

The uses of tissue culture are limited only by the imagination of the investigator (and the size of his grant funds). Cells can be fused and hybridized to make man-mouse combinations, or almost any other combination desired. In this manner genetic material is transferred and translocated, hundreds of gene sites are pinpointed precisely in the geography of the chromosomes, new genetic traits are imparted, and a truly marvelous repertoire of "genetic surgery" performed.

In tissue culture, cells can be punished to the limit—scalded, frostbitten, poisoned, loaded with allergens—in order to study the precise mechanisms of injury, and to test possible therapies for reversing or alleviating the damage. In fact, cell cultures provide an ideal testing ground for drugs of any kind, and have long been routinely used for this purpose. As one recent example: Allan L. Goldstein of the University of Texas Medical Branch (UTMB) at Galveston is co-discoverer of a hormone called thymosin, which we will hear more about later because it may turn out to be of some importance in aging. But its initial use has been in the treatment of inherited immune-deficiency diseases. When thymosin was deemed ready for clinical trials, there were two possible candidates for the first treatment. One was a boy in Houston who had lived in a plastic bubble for more than two years to keep him germ-free. The other was a girl in San Francisco who had been repeatedly hospitalized with recurring infections.

Any untried drug may (1) fail to work in human patients, or (2) cause adverse side effects. In the case of thymosin, animal studies had suggested it was relatively free of major hazards. Just the same, Goldstein and his collaborators were reluctant to use it on these children without some evidence, beyond the theoretical, that thymosin had a good chance of boosting their deficient immune systems. So they worked out a method for testing thymosin first in tissue culture. The Houston boy's cells did not form the telltale "rosette" shapes that indicate the production of immune cells (lymphocytes). This meant his bone marrow was not capable of manufacturing the incipient "stem cells" (perhaps because those genetic switches were mistakenly turned off) without which even thymosin cannot help the patient. (A possible alternative is a bone-marrow transplant.) There was no point in exposing the child to even a small additional risk. The cells of the San Francisco girl, however, responded with a strong display of rosettes, indicating that stem cells were present; her deficiency lay in an inability to convert them to mature lymphocytes. She was treated with thymosin, now gets a regular dose, and her infections seem to be well under control.

When the first anti-aging drugs are tested (and thymosin may be one of them), they will almost surely be tried initially *in vitro* to see if they can reverse the signs of aging in cultured cells.

But do cells truly age in culture? And, if so, is the process the same as *in vivo*? Does the study of cells in culture have anything at all to tell us about the physiological deterioration and death of human beings? Some think not. Among the more outspoken is Donner Denckla of the Roche Institute, creator of the best-worked-out hormonal-clock theory of aging (the "clock" being located in the brain). Denckla, originally an endocrinologist by trade and a relative newcomer to gerontology, says, "I don't care what happens to cells in tissue culture. What is important is *what people die of.*"

His own theory—a brilliant and promising one, based on experimental data as well as logic—will be dealt with at some length later in this book. In a word, he believes that the release of certain "death hormones" by the pituitary at scheduled times of life is what causes aging. Inasmuch as cells in tissue culture are beyond the reach of any hormonal influences (unless hormones are deliberately added to the culture), whatever "aging" seems to occur *in vitro* is an artifact, not related in any meaningful way to the real thing.

Stanford University's Leonard Hayflick, on the other hand, has founded the whole new discipline of "cytogerontology" (cellular aging) and has written papers bearing such titles as "Aging Under Glass." He firmly believes that the clock of aging lies within the nucleus of the individual cell. (In either case, the program is still genetically dictated.) Taking a stance directly opposite to Denckla's, Hayflick declares that "the primary causes of age changes can no longer be thought of as resulting from events occurring at the supracellular level, i.e., at cell hierarchies from the tissue level and greater. The cell is where the gerontological action lies. I believe therefore that purely descriptive studies done at the tissue, organ and whole animal level, as they pertain to the biology of aging, are less likely to yield important information on mechanism than studies done at the cell and molecular level."

Who is right? Is the clock of aging—if one exists—a single entity located in the brain which governs the aging and death of all cells? Or does each cell carry its own genetic clock? Which theory—if either—is compatible with what is observed both *in vitro* and *in vivo?* Are the two theories as incompatible with one another as they appear to be? Do they in any way encompass the ideas of competing aging theories?

When Hayflick first turned his attention to the life spans of cells *in vitro,* in the late 1950's and early 1960's, the prevailing belief was that cells in tissue culture could live on indefinitely. This belief, which ruled with the strength of dogma, had been mainly propagated by the experiments of the late Alexis Carrel of the Rockefeller Institute. Carrel, among his many real achievements—one of which earned him a Nobel prize—had long been credited with an erroneous one: the continuous maintenance, over a period of more than thirty-four years, of a culture of chick-heart fibroblasts (the embryonic cells that later give rise to connective tissue). Carrel put the first little sliver of embryonic heart in a flask in 1912. As the cells multiplied in their special medium in culture after culture, they were religiously tended over the remaining thirty-three years of Carrel's life and not permitted to die out for nearly another two years. The word "religiously" is used here only half as metaphor. The tending of the cells was very like a religious rite. In fact, everything in Carrel's lab took on this kind of ceremonial air as his celebrity grew. He even made his technicians carry out their solemn-high duties in flowing black robes with hoods. Though his theatricality was looked upon with distaste by many of his peers, he was an unquestionably great scientist; his data, and his interpretations of the data, were accepted without serious challenge. "From such experiments," says Morgan Harris, in *Cell Culture and Somatic Variation,* "came the widely heralded view of Carrel that tissue cells are potentially immortal if maintained as continuously proliferating strains *in vitro.*"

Hayflick, then working at the Wistar Institute in Philadelphia, where he did his trailbreaking experiments, did not set out to challenge Carrel at all. He and a colleague, Paul Moorhead, were trying to study the effects of cancer-causing viruses on normal cells in culture. "The single missing link in this research plan," he later recalled, on accepting the Robert W. Kleemeier Award of the Gerontological Society in 1973, "was the establishment of normal human cell cultures—a feat that, surprisingly, had not been satisfactorily accomplished in 1959. Since human tissue that is most easily available comes from operating theaters and is presumably abnormal, we turned to human embryonic tissue, not only because it represented presumptive normal tissue but because we reasoned that the likelihood of encountering unwanted latent viruses might also be reduced. . . .

"Until that time no one had determined that normal human cells could be cultured by invoking a wide variety of criteria including chromosome analysis. Prior to these studies normal human cells were only presumed to have been cultivated."

Why the long hiatus? Earlier, as Morgan Harris explains, "the methods at hand were too laborious for routine use, and the necessity for a complex, undefined medium prevented the application of analytical techniques. Owing to such limitations, cell culture had for many years relatively little general impact, and was regarded more as an art than as a basic research tool in biology and medicine." By the time Hayflick came onto the scene, the potential research uses of tissue culture had become much more widely recognized. The major surprise that grew out of his initial studies with Moorhead was "the finding that the normal cell populations grew and divided perfectly for many months, then slowed down, stopped dividing, and ultimately died."

As Hayflick repeatedly emphasizes, he was not the first to learn that normal cells in culture—unlike neoplastic strains—had a finite life span. Other researchers had made the same observation on numerous occasions, but nobody believed them. In fact, they often disbelieved their own results. Any contradiction of the Carrelian dogma was assumed to be due to the investigator's sloppiness; the cultures must have been contaminated. As we now know, it was Carrel's cultures that were contaminated. His technicians, as they kept adding fresh chick-embryo medium to maintain the cultures, did not realize that their "pure" medium also contained a few stray cells, which thus were being constantly, albeit inadvertently, added to the cultures. Once, at a meeting in Puerto Rico, Hayflick encountered one of Carrel's former technicians, who told him that she, for one, had been aware of what was happening but hadn't dared to say anything because so much was at stake!* Hayflick was more persistent than his predecessors. For one thing, he was certain, through repeated testing—as they perhaps could not have been—that he was working with a pure uncontaminated medium and with truly normal cells.

Hayflick's embryonic fibroblasts consistently underwent about fifty divisions (varying between forty and sixty "population doublings") before they reached what Hayflick calls "Phase III"—the point at which division ceases. Though this happens over a period of months *in vitro,* it could be an accelerated model of what requires all the years of a person's life *in vivo.* The figure of 50 ± 10 (50 plus or minus 10) doublings has become celebrated as "the Hayflick limit," and his favorite strain of fibroblasts, the WI-38† strain, widely used by others, has gained almost the same kind of fame in gerontological circles as the HeLa strain in cancer research. Once he had convinced himself that "the finite lifespan of cultured normal human and animal cells was a manifestation of biological aging at

* Last year, when Arthur Galston of Yale wrote a column about aging in *Natural History,* in which he repeated—as if it had never been challenged— Carrel's claims regarding the immortality of cells in culture, Hayflick, exasperated, dispatched a long letter and extracted an apology and retraction.
† WI for Wistar Institute, where they originated.

the cellular level," Hayflick decided to pursue cytogerontology as his central research interest. He has continued at Stanford* what he began at the Wistar Institute—where others, notably V. J. Cristofalo, have continued to do original work in the same field. Over the intervening years, Hayflick has performed many variations of his first experiments, and so have investigators in hundreds of laboratories around the world.

Before he ever submitted any of his data for publication, Hayflick wanted to reassure himself triply that his Phase III phenomenon did not come about because of some unsuspected fault in his culture medium—or through mere statistical wear and tear. It is easy, in cell clones, to distinguish male cells from female. Only female cells contain the so-called Barr bodies, which are clearly visible in the sex chromatin under a microscope. Hayflick grew out a pure male strain, let them divide until they had lived out most of their expected life spans, then added a pure young female strain to the culture. After the time when the male cells could be assumed to have arrived at Phase III, Hayflick carefully checked the culture and found that the viable cells were now 100 per cent female, still dividing vigorously on schedule. That clinched it. If there had been a contaminant present, it would not have discriminated against the male cells only, and left the female cells intact. It would have killed male and female alike, and the survivors, if any, should have included both sexes.

Hayflick submitted his carefully compiled report to *The Journal of Experimental Medicine,* which he considered to be "the Cadillac of medical journals" at the time. It was rejected and returned with what amounted to a kindly pat on the head. "The largest fact to have come out from [sic] tissue culture in the last fifty years," the editor wrote, "is that cells inherently capable of multiplying will do so indefinitely if supplied with the right milieu *in vitro.*" Though Hayflick usually neglects to mention it when he tells the story, the editor who signed the letter was Peyton Rous—whose own early work with the Rous chicken sarcoma virus had a similarly hard time gaining acceptance because everybody knew that viruses could not possibly cause cancer (another example of The Josh Billings Syndrome). Rous's discovery eventually won him a Nobel prize late in life, but

---

* In early 1976, Hayflick resigned his professorship at Stanford in a dispute that also involved NIH. The details are difficult to ascertain as this book goes to press, but the controversy appears to have no bearing on the nature or quality of Hayflick's research results.

it took a good many years—though he worked at the Rockefeller Institute—to make any headway among his peers. Yet Rous fell into the same trap which he had been victim of. This is, unfortunately, what typically happens to young revolutionaries in science, as in politics; they become old conservatives, who keep young revolutionaries from getting a proper hearing, not because they are ungenerous but through a failure of imagination.* (Hayflick did finally get his report published in *Experimental Cell Research*.)

As further evidence of a cellular aging program, Hayflick put cells in deep-frozen hibernation for long periods of time without affecting the Hayflick limit. In an ingenious series of experiments, a number of cultures were placed in storage at liquid nitrogen temperatures at varying "ages" (i.e., after a measured number of divisions); then thawed out, a few at a time, over a period of a dozen years. In each case, the cells "remembered" where their lives had been interrupted—say, at twenty divisions—and proceeded to double another thirty or so times before reaching Phase III.

Hayflick has also cited other evidence, based on work done in his own lab and in many others—especially by a diligent team of investigators headed by George M. Martin at the University of Washington School of Medicine in Seattle. When cell samples are taken from adults of varying ages, in general, the older they are the fewer times the cells divide before they attain Phase III. The cells of a twenty-year-old tend to have more "life" left in them, by this standard, than those of a fifty-year-old. The cells of even very elderly individuals still have a few doublings left, which—if the life of a cell *in vitro* up to Phase III can be considered a valid paradigm—suggests that people *rarely live out their potential life spans*.

In 1969, Samuel Goldstein of the McMaster University Medical Center in Hamilton, Ontario, cultured the cells of a child victim of progeria—the cruel disease that mimics speeded-up senescence—and found that they had only a few doublings left (like the cells of a very old man or woman) this side of Phase III. Other scientists, including the Seattle group as well as Robin Holliday in London, did similar experiments with the cells of people afflicted with genetic diseases that shorten the life span—Werner's syndrome, for example —and found that the cells' *in vitro* span was likewise shortened.

* These characteristics of older minds worry some people when they think about the prospects of prolongevity. But gerontologists hope that maintaining a more youthful physiology will also help keep the mental outlook "young."

Later Goldstein, who had done the work on the shortest-lived cells (progeria), carried out further experiments with cells that should be the longest-lived, those of the Galapagos tortoise. These were skin cells rather than embryonic cells, and the four strains Goldstein was able to use achieved from 72 to 144 doublings before Phase III—significantly more than the human limit. At other research centers, embryonic cells from chickens and mice were found to divide fewer times in culture than human cells do—but not as few as would be predicted from their proportional life spans. The data on the cells of other species is still too sparse to establish any definitive correlations.*

What else?

A number of experiments have been done in the "serial transplantation" of normal cells and tissues. As an animal ages, the tissue in question is transplanted to a younger animal (of the same carefully bred species, of course, to minimize chances of graft rejection); as that animal approaches senescence, the tissue is again transplanted to another young one. This goes on until the transplanted cells are no longer viable. The best known of these experiments was the series done by P. L. Krohn at the University of Birmingham with the skin cells of mice. Since then a variety of other cells have been serially transplanted, ranging from mammary tissues to lymphocytes and marrow cells—such as the well-known series carried out by David Harrison at the Jackson Laboratory.† In all these cases the cells lived longer than they would have in their original donors (long since dead), sometimes by as much as two or three lifetimes. But they all eventually died.‡

These serial-transplantation results have been pointed to by

* In fact, a study made in Australia in 1975, by Stanley, Pye, and MacGregor (*see bibliography*) failed to find any such correlations.

† The fact that cell lines transplanted from old mice functioned well in young animals, while young marrow did not noticeably improve deficiencies in aged mice, convinced Harrison that the aging of these cells could not be intrinsically timed but was rather dependent on the environment provided by the new host.

‡ This is still in dispute. One long-term lymphoid cell line has been kept going continuously in culture for some ten years now by Kurt Hirschhorn and his associates at the Mount Sinai Medical Center in New York. Critics of this kind of research insist that all such cell lines are contaminated by the Epstein-Barr virus and are therefore abnormal. Hirschhorn insists that, virus-contaminated or not, these cells are normal by standard criteria.

Hayflick's critics as evidence that he was wrong. Caleb Finch of the University of Southern California, citing Krohn's mouse-skin data, asked: If those cells had a built-in life span, why didn't they die on schedule? There must be some "youth factor," imparted to the cells by their new hosts, others reasoned, that extended their life spans. I was present at a meeting in Bar Harbor, Maine, where David Harrison was speaking. At one point, Robert Kohn—who was in the audience—said flatly to Harrison: "Your experiments have very neatly refuted Hayflick," and no one rose to refute Kohn.

Yet, to Hayflick, these transplantation findings serve as further confirmation of his cytogerontological thesis. He never claimed that "the Hayflick limit" *in vitro* applied to cells under other conditions. Obviously, human cells go through their *in vivo* lives at a much slower rate than they do in culture. The fact that transplantation increases the *duration* of a cell's life ("the passage of metabolic time") is interpreted by Hayflick and others—based on further experiments—as a slowing down of doublings.* Even if it were conclusively proven otherwise, Hayflick would not consider it any kind of refutation. He does not hold that there is no way to increase the life span; he is rather motivated by high hope that such ways will be discovered. To him, the fact of central importance which work such as Krohn's and Harrison's has demonstrated is that normal cells that have been carefully kept track of, growing not in culture but in the sites they normally occupy in the living body, *also* have finite life spans. In fact, when A. R. Williamson and B. A. Askonas of London's National Institute for Medical Research carried out serial transfers of an antibody-forming spleen-cell clone in mice, they proved to their own satisfaction that they had created a model demonstrating the limited life span of dividing cells *in vivo*. All this, in Hayflick's opinion, "circumvents arguments levelled at similar data obtained from the 'artificial' conditions of *in vitro* cell culture."

Critics eager to refute Hayflick find support in yet another, and quite different, set of experiments. These all involve the apparent extension of the cell's life span *in vitro* by adding various substances to the culture medium. Modest extensions of cellular life span (up to eighteen doublings beyond control cultures) have been achieved, for example, with cortisone and hydrocortisone by both A. Macieira-

---

* As Hayflick points out, he has deep-frozen cells for more than a dozen years before unthawing—thus fantastically "increasing their life spans," but not increasing the number of doublings.

Coelho in France and Cristofalo in Philadelphia. Why should this be so? It is known that the making of RNA as well as ribosomes (those protein-assembly workbenches again) decline as cells age. Macieira-Coelho and his colleague, E. Loria, speculate that cortisone and hydrocortisone may increase life span by maintaining the manufacture of ribosomes—and therefore of ribosomal RNA*—for longer periods of time. "It is interesting, however," as they note in their *Nature* report, "that when hydrocortisone is withdrawn from cells which have grown beyond the lifespan of the controls, the cultures die within two passages."

More recently and even more impressively, Berkeley's Lester Packer, in collaboration with James R. Smith of the Veterans Administration Hospital in Martinez, California, appears to have *doubled* cellular life spans by adding Vitamin E to the cultures. Ignoring the Hayflick limits of 50 ± 10 doublings, the cells thus treated went through 100 or more doublings without showing signs of abnormality. Moreover, they were still dividing vigorously when the experiment was terminated, so no maximum limit has yet been set for these revised conditions.

As I mentioned in the last chapter, antioxidants such as Vitamin E are believed to slow down oxidation reactions and combat free radical damage. Thus the Packer-Smith experiments (the results of which, it should be noted, are still in some dispute because others have had trouble duplicating them) would seem to lend strong support to Harman's free radical theory of aging. They would also seem to enhance the suspicion of Harman and others that the cell's mitochondria—the organelles that serve as energy machines to power the cell, and where most of the oxidation reactions therefore take place—are critical to the aging process. If indeed free radical damage is the principal cause of cellular aging *in vitro,* as the theory's proponents believe it to be *in vivo,* and if, further, the end result of the accumulated damage is the gradual cessation of cell division, then the Vitamin E experiments would be a truly dramatic demonstration—not only of the theory's validity, but of the powerful anti-aging potential of antioxidant therapy. But are such ideas consistent with observed events in tissue culture? Is there any evidence that free radical damage occurs at all *in vitro?* The evidence is indirect.

Certainly cells in culture do undergo a stage of fairly rapid deterio-

---

* The ingredient that went down so drastically in Strehler's aging beagles.

ration before they die, just as cells *in vivo* do. Hayflick's Phase III is not a clear-cut cellular event, a sudden cessation of all doubling at a precisely pinpointable moment. Even after all cells have stopped dividing—clearly beyond Phase III—"the culture," says Hayflick, "may linger for several weeks or months during which time the cells continue to degenerate to the point where they are all ultimately dead." Before the cells stop dividing altogether, the *rate* of division slows down, and the cells show many signs of senescence and the loss of vital functions. Even before the onset of this obviously degenerative pattern, biochemical tests can detect earlier signs of damage and deterioration. When these observations were first reported, they were taken as evidence that Orgel's error theory was correct. The work of Holliday in England and Macieira-Coelho in France particularly seemed to lend such support. "An error catastrophe process of this sort," wrote Macfarlane Burnet in *The Lancet,* "is the most likely interpretation of the cell-culture phenomenon known as the Hayflick limit"—though he expressed the belief that such errors came about through somatic mutations, under genetic control. The same results led others to the conclusion that the Hayflick limit was *not* built into the cell's genetics at all, but rather was a reflection of what statistics would lead one to expect when large numbers of cells, in artificial circumstances, were allowed to accumulate damage over long periods of time: gradual degeneration, the slowdown of division, the end of division, and eventual death. Denckla is among those who favor this interpretation; and Medvedev earlier predicted the likelihood of just such a statistical amassing of errors. Hayflick disagrees, of course—and feels that he convincingly refuted such charges in advance, before he ever published his first paper, by his careful studies in culturing male and female cell lines.

Nevertheless, further credence was lent to these interpretations by a series of experiments done at the State University of New York at Buffalo by a British-born team, James F. Danielli and Audrey Muggleton, using a relatively immortal species of amoeba. The basic question in cellular aging is the same *in vitro* as *in vivo:* Is it the nuclear DNA that dictates the running down of the cell's multifarious activities? Or is it rather a case of the cytoplasmic material—the protein-making machinery and the mitochondrial energy generators —finally, under the steady beatings that mere living entails, losing the capacity to follow the genetic orders? The Danielli-Muggleton results seemed to prove the latter. They transferred cytoplasmic material from a *mortal* species of amoeba to the cytoplasm of the immortal species—and, by so doing, conferred upon the immortals the gifts of old age and death!

But was the same true of human cells? Hayflick was eager to devise an experimental test that could provide an unequivocal answer. Working with his Stanford colleague Woodring E. Wright, with help from David Prescott of the University of Colorado, he devised an elaborate laboratory technique for enucleating cells en masse. There is a substance called cytochalasin B, extracted from mold, which can cause occasional cells to extrude their nuclei. Hayflick found he could considerably facilitate this process by spinning WI-38 cells in an ultracentrifuge until they were subjected to gravitational forces 25,000 times greater than the G force that keeps us on earth while it spins along in space. In a cell at 25,000 Gs, the nucleus migrates through the cytoplasm out to the membrane, where the cytochalasin B then pulls it the rest of the way through. Under these circumstances, some 99 per cent of the cells are enucleated. The remaining 1 per cent are rendered incapable of further division by treating them with mitomycin-C.

In other cells, again through a complex process, most of the enzymes in the cytoplasm could be inactivated by treatment with a poisonous substance, iodoacetate, while the nucleus generally remained intact. Then any two cells could be fused, using inactivated Sendai virus to bring about the fusion—a standard laboratory method. Employing such tools and techniques, Hayflick and Wright were able to join a young nucleus with an old cytoplasm, and vice versa, in diverse combinations and conditions. Carrying through numerous variations of these experiments, Hayflick and Wright found that, in every case, the number of doublings was dictated by the transplanted *nucleus*. If the nucleus of a cell which had already divided thirty times was placed in a very young cell, the resultant hybrid would divide only twenty or so times. On the other hand, if a fresh young nucleus—from a cell which had doubled, say, no more than ten times—was put into an enucleated cell almost ready for Phase III, it would then go on to divide another forty or so times before Phase III actually set in. Unlike the amoeba, then, the life span of the human cell does *not* seem to be affected by old cytoplasm. To double-check both his results and his interpretation of them, as well as the original amoeba experiments, Hayflick now has Audrey Muggleton working as a member of his Stanford team. But the hybridizing experiments already demonstrate beyond a reasonable doubt in his mind that the genetic aging program resides solely in the nuclear DNA.

Chapter VIII

DENCKLA: THE CLOCK IS
IN THE BRAIN

Even if Hayflick's interpretation—which I for one find most convincing—is accepted as correct, it resolves the debate only for those who believe that the clock of aging is located in the individual cell. It does not, of course, resolve anything for someone like W. Donner Denckla, for whom the clock of aging is hormonal in nature, and resides in the brain. There he sits, in his lab at Roche, a bespectacled, boyish-looking Harvard M.D., enthusiastic and brilliantly articulate. He exhorts, expounds, defends, refutes, gets up to pace and gesticulate, stops now and then to poke irritably at the large washtub-like vat with its complexity of glass tubing—a gadget of his own design for extracting the pituitary product he calls DECO (for "decreasing O_2 consumption" hormone) deliberately refraining from referring to it yet as "the death hormone," though others have not hesitated to do so. The gadget, which may well provide the most delicate hormone assays ever achieved and hence be applicable to Roche's other hormone work as well, is giving him some mechanical difficulties. He is impatient with the resulting holdup. He is still dissatisfied with the degree of purification he has been able to attain, but feels he is getting closer all the time.

Unlike Hayflick and most other gerontologists, Denckla does not have to worry about applying for grants each year. The Roche Institute of Molecular Biology—quite separate from the nearby research laboratories of Hoffmann LaRoche, Inc., though also supported by that enlightened pharmaceutical house—maintains a campus-like atmosphere, where scientists are encouraged to pursue their own research without regard to any practical payoff, and may

66

also publish their findings freely. Denckla does not, of course, get *all* the support he would like; but he is relieved of the frustrating, time-consuming chore of writing new grant proposals, and the necessity to keep re-justifying his existence.

Denckla's belief in a brain-based hormonal clock of aging is supported by the similar views of USC's Caleb Finch, who is convinced that one or more hormones must play a large part in aging, and that certain small areas of the brain must be an important part of the clockwork. Also sympathetic to this outlook is James Bonner of Caltech, and a few of Bonner's graduate students, most notably Mahlon Wilkes. I was on hand in Bonner's lab one late afternoon when he was preparing to leave for Mahlon Wilkes's house in Pasadena, where the first meeting of a small, newly formed aging-research group was to be held. The group consisted mainly of graduate students from both USC and Caltech, surrounding the two principal figures, Bonner and Finch. Though Bonner is the senior man, he is more the molecular biologist whose long interest in the mechanisms of genetic on-off switching has brought him to gerontology; whereas Finch considers himself to be a dedicated gerontologist. In any case, Bonner voluntarily took a side seat, and it was the younger Finch who presided. The group was, well, not exactly *anti*-Hayflick, but certainly non-Hayflick, in its orientation. And they might be described as pro-Denckla, except that at this point it seemed to me they were insufficiently familiar with Denckla's more recent experiments and conclusions to center on him as the symbol of their own investigative thrust.

Earlier, a little farther down the coast, I had discussed Denckla's ideas with Roger Guillemin at the Salk Institute in La Jolla, who seemed startled to hear that someone was already actively trying to isolate "death hormones." His own research group had been thinking along the same lines, but so far had had no opportunity to pursue the hunch further. But it all made excellent sense to him. Guillemin believes, however, that if death hormones are released by the pituitary, this release is in turn triggered by "releasing factors" in the hypothalamus—a sequence which now appears to be true for *all* hormones secreted by the pituitary. (This is the area Guillemin has pioneered so fruitfully.) Denckla agrees Guillemin may be right; if so, it still leaves his theory intact—and more hopeful in the long run, since releasing factors are smaller, simpler, and therefore easier to synthesize than pituitary hormones. Nathan Shock, too, at a recent Miami meeting, cited data which suggested to him that aging "must be regarded as a breakdown of endocrine and neural control mechanisms." Looking at what he considered to be the limitations of cellular-aging theories such as Hayflick's, Shock urged that more attention be given to what happens to the total organism.

Similar views have been espoused quite vigorously for some time in the U.S.S.R., especially by V. V. Frolkis, who works at Chebotarev's Institute of Gerontology in Kiev. "The aging of an organism," writes Frolkis in *The Main Problems of Soviet Gerontology,* "is not a simple sum of aging of its individual cells. At each new level of biologic organization appear not only quantitative but also qualitative features of the aging process. That's why the analysis of the neuro-humoral regulation (brain, nerves, glands, hormones) adapting the activity of cells to the needs of the whole organism, is of primary importance for the purpose of understanding the essence of aging of a whole organism."

If the endocrine system is so heavily involved, is there, then, a "master gland" for aging? Sir Macfarlane Burnet had nominated the thymus, which controls the immunological surveillance system; and this view gained considerable support from the work of Allan Goldstein in Galveston with the thymic hormone, thymosin—though Bar Harbor's David Harrison has pointed out a number of key experiments which cast doubt on the thymus as an intrinsically timed aging mechanism in itself. For similar reasons and others of his own, Donner Denckla prefers to regard the thyroid as the critical gland in aging—apart from the pituitary itself, which governs all the other endocrine glands. This is a belief he has arrived at through logic as well as experiment. After much study of autopsy data and death records, Denckla finds that people—in fact, all mammals—die through the failure of one of two major body systems: the cardiovascular or the immune system. (This assumes that cancer is an immunological disease, as more and more researchers deem it to be. If this assumption proves wrong, cancer will have to be added as a third major cause of death.)

Denckla points out that people do not really die of heart failure, or kidney failure, or liver malfunction, or stroke; these are merely the end results of the failure either of the immune cells to do their job or of the blood vessels to deliver oxygen and nutrients where they are needed. There is only one gland that has a profound effect on both systems—the thyroid. Finch, too, has suggested that "a key candidate for a central endocrine change of aging . . . is the thyroid, whose obligatory role in central, autonomic, and endocrine functions is well documented."

Approaching the problem from another vantage point, Denckla carefully studied data on many species of animals, and found a fairly consistent correlation among five biological time periods: the heart rate, the metabolic rate, the time of gestation (specially defined), the time to puberty, and the time from puberty to death. In all these timed events, Denckla believes, the thyroid gland is of central importance because its product, thyroxine, is *the master rate-controlling hormone* for *all cells and tissues.* It governs the basal metabolic rate, the speed at which cells burn their fuel and consume their oxygen.

Moreover, says Denckla, the disease which most closely mimics premature aging in adults is hypothyroidism. It can be fatal if untreated, and the victim is more susceptible to infection, which suggests a diminished immune capability. We almost never see advanced cases of hypothyroidism these days, because thyroxine is prescribed as soon as a deficiency is discovered. But in the 1890's, when thyroxine was first administered, the reversals were quite dramatic: wrinkles disappeared, gray hair turned black or brown or blond again, resistance to disease returned to normal levels. Encouraged by these results, doctors used thyroxine to reverse the symptoms of aging in the really old. But the treatment quickly went out of style because (1) it didn't work, and (2) the high dosage killed some of the patients. Denckla's own work sheds light on the reasons for this outcome.

Though Denckla is an analytical theorist, he bases his theories on experiments with more than 2,500 rats of varying ages, some normal, some without ovaries, some without pancreases, some without adrenals, and so on. He has measured the metabolic rates of anesthetized animals under the most rigorously controlled conditions, making carefully computed adjustments for body weight, fat content, and other circumstances. He was able to ascertain that only the pituitary or thyroid make a difference in the metabolic rate (the thyroid being controlled by the pituitary), and that the pituitary slows down the metabolic rate with age, not by failing to stimulate the thyroid to make its hormones, but rather by releasing a blocking hormone (DECO, the death hormone?) that prevents the cells from properly using the thyroxine that still freely circulates in the animal's bloodstream.

Denckla has since ascertained that aging men and women—if they are normal, not hypothyroid—are not short of thyroxine either. Plenty of it circulates in the bloodstream, but the cells somehow cannot take it up and use it. Denckla believes that, in people as in rats, the pituitary gland begins at puberty to release the first of a series of those death hormones—Finch calls them "anti-thyroid hormones"—which act at the cell membrane to keep thyroxine out.* These are the hormones he is trying so hard to isolate, purify and synthesize. It is interesting to note, in this context, that V. V. Frolkis has reported the presence of increased concentrations in the blood, with age, of substances that *do* inhibit the functioning of pancreatic hormones—much as Denckla believes his DECO inhibits the functioning of thyroid hormone. Frolkis quite independently notes the decline, with age, of the blood's ability to bind thyroxine!

A diminished supply of thyroxine within the cell would cause a number of critical imbalances. These imbalances could bring on— or at least allow the onset of—the destructive changes we associate with the aging process. Oxidation may be speeded up, creating more free radicals, thus more cross-linkages, more mutations, more error catastrophes. More toxins may be produced, leaving more cellular garbage than the cell can dispose of. Immune cells, too, become less efficient, sometimes attacking other cells, creating autoimmune phenomena, and adding to the general disruption. The death hormone may act on the thymus cells to cut down production of

* In late 1975, Denckla told me of new experimental results just being prepared for publication at the time, which reinforced his convictions by restoring certain cardiovascular and immunological functions to aging animals. In the blood vessels of aging rats, total peripheral resistance goes down three- or four-fold, and the "beta" receptors (responsible for vascular relaxation and dilatation) virtually disappear. Meanwhile, the immune system's phagocytic activity—the characteristic engulfment of foreign material—goes down by five- or six-fold, and T-cell immunity to a lesser extent.

Denckla was able to "restore juvenile competence" in all these areas by (1) removing the pituitary (the presumed source of DECO) and (2) administering thyroxine! Giving thyroxine to animals with intact pituitaries had no rejuvenating effect at all.

A few weeks later, he was able to report that youthful levels of the enzyme RNA polymerase in the liver—which goes down about four-fold with age in the rat—had also been restored, demonstrating that thyroxine was operating at the genetic level.

thymosin (perhaps even causing the shrinkage of the thymus that occurs in everyone at a relatively early age), further impairing immunologic function and increasing the risk of cancer and lethal infection. The death hormones might even operate principally at the level of genetic on-off switching. As Finch has pointed out, "hormones influence cellular activities at both the nuclear and cytoplasmic levels of control."

Medvedev once postulated a built-in genetic death mechanism, and Howard Curtis even hypothesized the existence of death hormones, but he took it no farther than the raw suggestion. There is nothing inconsistent in the idea that death hormones, if they exist, could be responsible for aging changes in all the varieties of both dividing and nondividing cells. The DNA in the original fertilized egg does in fact program all the body's cells to perform their astonishing multiplicity of tasks. Thus groups of differently programmed cells, which have already lived out radically different lives, may also "know how" to die differently. In a well-trained army—with units of infantry, artillery, cavalry, tank corps, air support, all ready to go—the commanding general does not have to issue specific detailed instructions an hour before the battle. All he needs to do is give the prearranged signal, and the pre-programmed units all speed to their diverse and unique tasks—though coordinated by the original battle plan. A death or aging hormone could, in a similar manner, command legions of cells to perform separate actions. It would not have to *cause* the specific detailed changes; it would simply *trigger* the sequences of events already pre-programmed in the given cell. "The high level of adaptation of the organism," as Frolkis reminds us, "has been reached in the process of evolution due to the *centralization of the processes of regulation* [italics supplied], the centralization which on the one hand made it possible to unite the activity of individual cells, organs and systems in achieving a common adaptive effect and on the other hand to ensure within certain limits a degree of autonomy of their metabolism and functions against the background of these centralized reactions."

In Denckla's tidy scheme, however, at least one important question remains unanswered: How to account for the running out of genetic program in cells in Hayflick cultures, which are certainly beyond the reach of any brain-based hormonal clock of aging? If Hayflick is right, can Denckla be? The two views seem irreconcilable. That's why proponents of hormonal theories are so often affronted by Hayflick's findings, and have felt it necessary to question the data or to minimize their meaning. The same has been true of Denckla.

But Denckla may have inadvertently supplied an answer of sorts. On many occasions I have questioned him in his lab at Roche, or while pacing before his blackboard at home in Tenafly. During these conversations he has often returned to the matter of why, to him, it makes so much sense to assume an underlying genetic program (an assumption he shares with Hayflick and so many others) that sets the limit to how long any individual of a given species can live.

Denckla's reasoning (in inchoate form, at least, it dates back as far as August Weismann in the late nineteenth century) goes something like this: The environment keeps changing as time goes on. (It changes more for land mammals than for sea creatures.) In order to adapt to these changes, the species must evolve in favorable ways through genetic mutations. But evolution is a slow process. As the environment changes, there must be a sufficiently rapid turnover of generations to allow those characteristics best fitted for the changed conditions to be incorporated into the gene pool. Whether the population consists of pinworms, pterodactyls, or people, species survival requires a large enough quantity of individuals in any given generation to ensure that a significant number of them will be the beneficiaries of chance mutations that can be passed along, and a short enough life span to permit the necessary turnover. As Jonas Salk puts it in *Survival of the Wisest,* "Even though Death eventually wins over Life as far as the individual is concerned, Life wins over Death in the perpetuation of the species."

Thus Denckla believes there must exist "an absolutely fail-safe killing mechanism without which the species would not survive." Now, a fail-safe system in rocketry or weaponry means redundancy —backup systems that will take over in case the primary system fails to function. So it may be with our program for aging and death. Suppose Denckla is right, and the release of specific death hormones is the primary self-destruct mechanism. The cellular aging program could be a *backup* system, designed to set a second limit, in case the death hormones somehow fail to be released, or to be effective. Finally, if all else fails, wear and tear alone would do the job.

As Hayflick has suggested, "normal cells have a finite capacity for replication, and . . . this finite capacity is rarely if ever reached by cells *in vivo,* but when freed of *in vivo* constraints can be reached *in vitro.*" Hayflick's suggestion is borne out by the conclusions of the noted German pathologist Ludwig Aschoff, who wrote, in 1938, after long observation and hundreds of autopsies (the quote is from a paper by Finch): "It is my conviction that natural death in human beings never occurs, or only in rare instances. Autopsies which have been made on the very old always show a pathological cause. In life the severe disease changes of those advanced in years are usually not felt. When I visited a 97-year-old man two days before his death, he showed so little the symptoms of a serious illness that I was convinced on hearing of his demise that at last I had seen a case of natural death. I was very surprised when I found at the autopsy stipulated by the deceased, a severe lobar pneumonia of at least four to five days' duration and numerous metastases from a malignant tumor of the thyroid gland. The old man had diagnosed none of these disorders in himself, although he was well equipped by training to do so and had carefully observed himself."

Aschoff's comments recall Denckla's impatience with what happens to cells *in vitro.* "I care what people *die of.*" And what they die of are the *"in vivo* constraints" to which Hayflick refers. One can imagine that if Denckla's research were ever to result in the successful removal of those *in vivo* constraints—perhaps by preventing the release of death hormones—we might after all be in deadly danger from the cessation of division in, say, our skin or gut cells. If we solved that, we would still have wear-and-tear damage to contend with—which seems a formidable undertaking, though it might be less so if we learn to keep the repair genes switched on so the cell can simply continue to maintain the integrity of its systems indefinitely.

The idea that the cellular aging program might be a redundant, fail-safe backup system for a hormonal aging program is further bolstered, in my own view, by still another set of Denckla's own experimental and theoretical considerations.

In his experiments with those thousands of rats, it was important for Denckla to develop the most meticulous possible set of metabolic measurements he could devise. Instead of the usual basal metabolic rate (BMR)—also known as the resting oxygen consumption rate—Denckla evolved a finer measure which he called MOC for *minimum* oxygen consumption rate. He was thus able to pin down the specific thyroid-influenced component which accounted for the steep drop in metabolic rate with aging. He was also able to discern, separately, a much lower, much steadier "athyroidal component" of the metabolic rate, which was not affected by the presence or absence of thyroid hormone. This was essentially the same rate as that measured in animal tissues *in vitro*. Denckla calls this component the GMR, the *genetic* metabolic rate. Unlike the MOC, which is controlled by the endocrine centers of the brain, the GMR is controlled by the individual cell's DNA.

Thus it would appear that the MOC is a reflection of the brain-based clock of aging at work, while the GMR could well be the medium through which Hayflick's cellular clock operates in those WI-38 cultures. In the one case, the cells in the brain responsible for hormonal release are turned *on* at the appropriate times; in the other case, the genetic information required to keep the cell machinery functioning is gradually turned *off*. In both cases, it looks as if we come back to the on-off switching mechanisms in the DNA of individual cells. If all this be so, then Denckla is right—and Hayflick is also right. And Strehler too. And Harman, and Orgel, and Burnet, and practically everyone else. At least it would appear that their theories aren't *wrong,* just incomplete.

Yet another possibility is that the clock of aging in the brain and the clock of aging in the cell (if either—or both—exist) are not really separate programs at all, but rather a single, delicately orchestrated program; and that, under the unnatural circumstances of tissue culture, that part of the program which resides in the DNA of the individual cells expresses itself in an unprogrammed solo performance—or perhaps a smaller group performance, much as say, a violin section, isolated from the main body of the orchestra as well as the conductor, could still play out its score, uninterrupted by any on-off signals from the conductor, from the beginning to the end.

Whether Hayflick or Denckla turns out to be right, or if neither of them does, one can still see the coming together of data and ideas in overarching concepts that incorporate many diverse theories of aging: genetic switching, cross-linkage, free radicals, autoimmunity, somatic mutations, error catastrophes. V. V. Frolkis has pointed out dryly that "the number of hypotheses is generally inversely proportional to the clarity of the problem." Now, with hypotheses fast converging, the problem has obviously taken an encouraging turn in the direction of clarity.

Chapter IX

HEREDITY AND
IMMUNITY

Like Denckla, Macfarlane Burnet believes that aging and death "are essential to the evolutionary process, and the age at which they happen must be related to the life style of the species concerned." Yet many gerontologists, even those who lean favorably toward a genetic aging program (Strehler and Orgel, for example), have been reluctant to accept the idea that evolutionary necessity has dictated the precise control of the aging process. What, they ask, is the evolutionary advantage of programming organisms to deteriorate and die at such relatively advanced ages?

Evolution, they agree, must indeed have programmed us (much as the space engineers program their planetary fly-bys) to survive in reasonable health and vigor until our job is done—i.e., until we have sired, borne, and reared the next generation; otherwise we wouldn't be here to argue the matter. But positive programming for propagation is not the same as the building in of self-destruct mechanisms to guarantee aging and death at specified times. Is it not rather a case of simply abandoning the machine and letting it run down (again, like the planetary fly-by)? If the Pacific salmon's machine begins to run down within days of spawning, so be it. If the human machine takes some years to run down, so be it also.

Back in 1941, the late J. B. S. Haldane argued—in *New Paths in Genetics*—that evolution would be unlikely to select either for or against mutations that occurred in individuals after their reproductive lives were over. Even so, Finch speculates that our aging patterns may still be there in the genes that were selected in the past for whatever advantages they may have bestowed earlier in

75

life, in terms of reproduction and species survival. In this scheme, aging would still be accidental, but genetically programmed nevertheless.

Suppose an automotive engineer wanted to design a car that would get off to a very fast start; to give it the necessary horsepower, he might have to supply an engine that could achieve speeds up to 150 or 200 miles per hour—far faster, perhaps, than the driver would ever intend to go. An innocent bystander who had no knowledge or insight into the engineer's problems might well say, "Why would anyone have built a car capable of going 150 or 200 miles an hour if that's not what he had in mind?" If no one knew how fast the car would go, and no one had ever tried driving it faster than, say, 60 mph—and then a new and more adventurous driver came along and decided to test the car to its limit, he would discover that the "programmed" velocity was two or three times greater than previously believed. In fact, the "program" had nothing to do with the car's ultimate speed limit, but only with getting the car off to a fast start.

Thus evolutionary nature may not have intended that any living creatures survive much past their reproductive days or years. It could rely on mere exposure to environmental hazards and stresses, including predators and infectious organisms, to end their lives quickly once their primary mission, procreation, was accomplished. Human organisms, it's true, require many years of nurture by parents or guardians before they reach adulthood; yet, in ancient times, an average life expectancy of well under thirty years was enough to ensure the turnover of generations which Denckla's theory requires.

In the wild it is hard to find any living specimens of aging animals; nevertheless, their species thrive. Even domestic animals, protected as they are from the major dangers of wear and tear and predation, are not protected from us, their protectors, and we usually butcher them before senescence gets a chance to set in. Yet, as all zookeepers know, wild animals do grow old in captivity. And domestic animals show all the signs of senescence when they are permitted to live long enough—as Dr. Mike Tumbleson has demonstrated on his farm for aging pigs at the University of Missouri. Only a gerontological farm could afford to operate on this basis. It obviously would make no economic sense for an ordinary farmer to keep feeding animals for years and years after their peak of productivity and marketability had been attained. There are, of course, rare exceptions such as the thoroughbred race horse who has won a sufficient number of purses to entitle him to a few years of serene pasturing. And most of us have seen our pets grow old and die.

We accept that all organisms—whether we can find aged specimens or not—do age eventually; and that, barring accidents, they age at a rate that is roughly "species-specific." This universal fact seems, after all, to throw the odds in the direction of Denckla's fail-safe mechanism. If organisms were really on their own without such a specific aging mechanism, suppose they were lucky and survived for indefinitely long periods of time (as indeed the planetary fly-bys are likely to, out in the vacuum of space); in that case, the earth might soon run out of room for newcomers with fresh genetic combinations. One can readily see that such an eventuality might be anti-evolutionary in its effects.

Hayflick would probably agree that evolution has built in a genetic aging mechanism—except, as we know, in regard to its location. Daniel Dykhuizen of the Australian National University in Canberra, goes along with Hayflick's conclusion that (in Dykhuizen's words): "cell senescence itself, rather than senescence of the organism, is the genetically controlled and programmed event selected by evolution," and that senescence at the level of the total organism is a reflection of what happens in myriads of that organism's individual cells. Dykhuizen puts forth, in *Nature,* a fascinating theory to explain how the cellular clock permits cells to proliferate when necessary, as in wound healing, yet turns off division at other times—for instance, to limit the growth of the damaging plaques that form on the walls of arteries. He challenges the idea that the random accumulation of errors in cells can alone account for senescence, again, on the same grounds as Hayflick: the failure of "transformed" (abnormal or malignant) cells to age and die under the same circumstances. As we saw in the last chapter, this exceptional behavior is as true *in vivo* as *in vitro.* When normal skin cells or lymphocytes are transplanted from one animal to another—even to a younger one of the same breed—they might live longer than otherwise, but they do die out, while cancer cell lines go on and on.

Roy Walford believes we may have something very important to learn about aging from transformed cells. Such cells are usually thought of as being cancerous, or at least pre-cancerous. Walford admits they are surely abnormal and even that they have taken the first step in the direction of malignancy. But the fact that they have taken this first step does not imply that the next step is inevitable—especially if the mechanism of transformation is under our own control. His daring proposal is that we deliberately seek to transform cells this first step of the way, but to stop the process right there.

Cells are already routinely transformed *in vitro,* usually by means of viruses, in order to study the process by which normal cells turn into cancer cells. But this is done mainly for the purpose of learning how to *prevent* transformation from occurring in the human body. Walford is suggesting that we make it come about by design; but not to apply this knowledge, of course, until we have also learned to forestall the cell's continuing transformation to a state of uncontrollable malignancy.

The idea of deliberately rendering healthy cells abnormal may seem bizarre, but only until we consider that the goal of gerontology is exactly that: to free ourselves of the normality that is senescence. If we can in fact turn on those genes which the clock of aging has turned off—or keep specific aging genes from being turned on, if that is the way it works—and if we can do it without producing cancer as a result, we will perhaps have gone a long way toward thwarting the genetic fail-safe mechanism, and thus bestowed upon our cells the same relative immortality which transformed cells enjoy.

Even if we could do what Walford proposes, the solution would seem to apply only to dividing cells. What of those all-important cells—the ones whose loss of function is, indeed, more likely to kill us—that have stopped dividing? The fact that mitotic and postmitotic cells are so basically different in this respect does not preclude a single aging mechanism for both. "There are two schools of thought in gerontological research," as Hayflick explains in *Medical World News.* "One says we age because our cells that divide have lost that ability, so there's a loss of numbers; the other says we age because the cells that don't divide, like neurones and muscle cells, lose their functional capacity over a long period. But that's a false distinction, because the division capacity of cells *is* a function. So it's the *decrement of function,* whether it be manifest as loss of doubling, loss of making enzymes, of what have you, that may affect aging."

The genes that stop division, then, may be the same genes that trigger aging in nondividing cells as well. What makes Walford hopeful about his suggestion is the belief that the transformation might be achieved by tampering with no more than *three or four genes on a single chromosome*. At least, that is the situation in mouse chromosomes, and Walford feels there is good reason for assuming the same is probably true in human cells.

Inasmuch as Walford's name, like Burnet's, is mainly associated with the immunological theory of aging, we might expect him to select the genes involved in immunological control to be in control of aging as well. Walford never did claim that the immune theory, as originally proposed, was the total explanation for human aging—especially in terms of causation. But now he feels that immune function and dysfunction, taken together with the built-in genetic controls as an added theoretical ingredient, can account for so many of the phenomena observed in the laboratory that it might well be the major cause of aging. This fits well with Burnet's comment in *The Lancet:* "If there is any reasonably simple clue to the nature of aging there must at some point be a nexus between information in the genome [the genetic manual of instructions] and some key process in the organism which sets the tempo of the ageing process." (Burnet's guess at the time [1973] was that the nexus lay in the configuration of key enzymes associated with DNA replication and repair.)

The immune theory originally dealt principally with *auto*immunity, the immune system's propensity for attacking the body's own tissues. But that is only part of the story. The other part—as evidenced by a series of experiments carried out by Ian C. Roberts-Thomas and his associates at Australia's Walter and Eliza Hall Institute and Royal Melbourne Hospital—is that the protective immunological response is consistently lower in old people than in young adults; and that in groups of old people of similar ages but differing immune responses, the highest mortality occurs in those with least immunity. Experiments the world over—in Walford's lab at UCLA, in Burnet's at Melbourne, in Makinodan's at NIH; by E. J. Yunis and his associates at the University of Minnesota, and by Robert A. Good's team at the Memorial Sloan-Kettering Cancer Institute in New York, to name a few—have yielded similar results, which, oversimplified, can be expressed in two statements:

1. As the organism ages, the protective efficiency of the immune system goes *down*.

2. As the organism ages, the autoimmune responses go *up*.

It is as if the armed forces of a constantly beleaguered community (which fairly describes a human body in the real world) were to grow increasingly careless about keeping out or hunting down invading forces, who were thus free to destroy and despoil at will and, at the same time, began to attack their own fellow citizens. In that event, the formerly secure population suddenly finds itself set upon simultaneously by both the cops and the robbers!

There could be no more literal self-destruct mechanism than programming the body's most efficient destroyer cells to attack the body's "civilian" cells. Autoimmune responses now seem to account for much more than those diseases officially recognized as being of autoimmune origin. A series of studies carried out by two members of Roberts-Thomas's Hall Institute team (Senga Whittingham and Ian R. Mackay), in collaboration with J. D. Matthews of Oxford's Radcliffe Infirmary, strongly suggest that autoimmunity is a major factor in the development of atherosclerosis, hypertension, and other degenerative diseases of aging. Roy Walford was able to extend the life span of mice by administering high doses of immunosuppressive drugs that effectively lowered immune response. Seymour Gelfand and J. Graham Smith, Jr., of the Medical College of Georgia at Augusta, in considering why cortisone and hydrocortisone had "released from aging" cells *in vitro,* suggested that the immunosuppressive capacity of these drugs had been responsible. The trick, of course, is to lower autoimmunity without at the same time lowering the aging animal's ability to resist infection.

Some success has been reported in this area, too. For instance, Makinodan challenged the immune systems of young mice by exposing them to bacteria. He then injected their lymphocytes into old mice who were, as a result, able to resist lethal doses of the same strain of bacteria for many months. He has suggested that the day might arrive when human beings could deposit goodly stores of lymphocytes in the deepfreeze while their immune systems are young and at their productive peak, then draw on them for support when they grow old. Such cells, in addition to being healthy and active, would presumably be free of autoimmune "memories" that the body's aging lymphocytes may have developed in the intervening years.

Further support for the immune theory of aging—especially that aspect of it which regards immune *deficiency* as being of critical importance—comes from the results of experiments done with a short-lived breed of dwarf mice which, as part of their inherited short-comings, are handicapped by low levels of immunity. To raise their immune levels, N. Fabris of the EURATOM Unit at Italy's University of Pavia, working with W. Pierpaoli and E. Sorkin of the Albert Schweitzer Research Institute at Davos-Platz, Switzerland, gave the dwarf mice injections of lymph-node lymphocytes. As a result, they were able to double—in some cases, almost triple—the life expectancies of their subjects. Fabris, Pierpaoli, and Sorkin believe that the lowered immunity, and therefore the shortened life span, of these mice is due to genetic *endocrine* deficiency. They argue convincingly that an intimate and necessary link exists between hormones and the proper activation and functioning of the immune system. It is in fact through immunological advances (pre-Denckla) that we have probably become most aware of the role that hormones may play in aging.

We have long been familiar with the phenomenon of immunity and have made practical use of its principles through a variety of medications and vaccines. Yet it is only in the past twenty years that we have come to any real understanding of what those principles are and how the immune system works. The last decade especially has produced an explosive acceleration in our acquisition of immunological knowledge. To appreciate how hormones and immunity are related, and what this relationship has to do with the aging process, requires at least a minimal grasp of immune mechanisms; this minimal understanding is all I shall attempt to convey*:

The key to human immunity lies in the small white blood cell called the *lymphocyte*. The normal adult human body contains something like 1 trillion lymphocytes, and about 10 million of these are being replaced by new ones every minute of every day—at least until the organism arrives at the early stages of the aging process. Lymphocytes appear to originate mainly in the bone marrow as immature "stem cells."

Large quantities of these, perhaps as many as half or more, mature directly into the bloodstream and are called B-lymphocytes or B-cells. The main function of B-cells is the manufacture of *anti-*

* Omitted from this account, for instance, is the remarkable advance in our understanding of antibodies, based on such research as that by Nobel biologist Gerald Edleman of Rockefeller University.

bodies—proteins whose major function is to fight bacterial infections. The body's B-cells* are encoded to recognize some 10,000 different potential invading substances (antigens). Once a B-cell is challenged by a foreign antigen, it starts to make antibodies to combat that specific antigen. From then on, it keeps making only that antibody and no other, and its descendants inherit the capacity to make the same antibody and to recognize the same antigen. That's one reason why immunological memory can last so long.

The rest of the lymphocytes pass through the thymus, and for that reason are called T-lymphocytes or T-cells. The thymus, the pinkish-gray mass located just behind the breastbone and just below the neck, shrinks to insignificant size early in life. Its function had always been anybody's guess, and modern doctors tended to look upon it as another useless vestigial organ, like the appendix. In fact, there was an unfortunate period in this century when doctors deliberately shrunk, by irradiation, thymuses mistakenly believed to be "enlarged." But all that was changed by the ingenious research of several investigators working independently of one another—notably Sloan-Kettering's Robert Good, then at the University of Minnesota, and Jacques Miller at England's Chester Beatty Research Institute (now at Australia's Hall Institute). Their experiments clearly established the thymus gland's importance in the body's defense system. Moreover, it soon became evident that *all* lymphoid tissue (which is where the lymphocytes live when they're not circulating) plays a role in immunity—including even the tonsils, adenoids, and appendix!

But the thymus turned out to be the "master gland of immunity,"† which is why Burnet, one of the fathers of the immunological theory of aging, proposed the thymus as the master gland of aging as well. In agreement with him, as a result of their dwarf mice studies, were the Italian-Swiss team of Fabris, Pierpaoli, and Sorkin. "Because the immunological function is fundamental for survival," they wrote in *Nature,* "if its function declines before other body functions, it would be a major determinant in the ageing processes.

---

* The B in B-cells does not stand for either bacteria or blood. Because, in the chicken, these cells were first found to be located in the bursa, their human counterparts were named "bursa-equivalent," or B for short.
† A baby born without a thymus is a child essentially without immunity—though such a child, if his bone marrow is capable of making stem cells, still can have B-cells and thus manufacture antibodies.

"We emphasize here the possible importance of the thymus as a biological clock and of hormones for the ageing process of the lymphoid system. We evaluate the capacity of lymphocytes, whose formation depends on hormones, to prevent early death and ageing processes." As we have seen, lymphocytes were able to postpone aging and death in the dwarf mice. "The full development of the thymus and the thymus-dependent lymphoid cells which can be induced by hormonal treatment in the post-weaning period," they continued, "results in the prevention of early ageing and considerable prolongation of life. . . . Therefore we wish to propose with Burnet that the thymus might be considered as an important organ for ageing control of body tissues. One could predict then that the longer the thymus functions at its optimal level either as producer of humoral factors and/or lymphocytes, the longer will be the life-span."

The T-cell, then, merits our special attention. A lymphocyte that passes through the thymus to become a T-cell does not make antibodies at all. It becomes, instead, a hand-to-hand combat specialist. Whereas B-cells use antibodies as their chemical weapons, T-cells act as assault troops. They attack, surround, destroy, ingest, or in one way or another inactivate the invaders. Because they do act in this direct manner, the T-cell function is called "cell-mediated immunity," in contrast to the B-cell antibody "humoral immunity" system. This is the kind of immunity involved in rejecting transplanted tissue and in killing cancer cells.

Many immunologists now believe what Burnet's fertile intellect, again, first hypothesized: that one class of lymphocytes is constantly carrying out an "immunological surveillance" of all the body's cells. As soon as a cell becomes malignant or even shows signs of pre-malignant changes, the T-cell scavengers move in before it can begin multiplying. (Thus, before Walford's scheme to transform cells on purpose could become workable, there would be another problem to overcome: how to protect them from being destroyed by the body's immune system? But this problem must be dealt with in any case if we are to overcome the body's natural increase in autoimmune response as it ages.) It makes sense, then, that, as thymus function declines with age, immune function also declines—and the incidence of cancer goes up.

While all this was being worked out in many laboratories and in many theorizing minds around the world, a team of scientists at the

National Cancer Institute conducted a critical experiment: Into a newborn baby mouse without a thymus, they implanted thymus tissue. But they put the tissue into a container with holes too small for a lymphocyte (or anything else of cell size) to get out. In spite of this barrier, *something* got through those tiny holes to stimulate the spleen and lymph nodes into making their own lymphocytes. That something almost had to be a hormone; and if that were the case, then the thymus was proven to be an endocrine gland.

Before 1960 such a hormone had not even been suspected. Now it became apparent that if a hormone released by the thymus could induce stem cells to mature into lymphocytes, then going through the thymus itself was not necessary after all. Thus, if a child were born without a thymus, or if a patient later had to lose his (the thymus is sometimes removed as a therapeutic measure in, for instance, myasthenia gravis), possession of the hormone alone might serve as an adequate substitute. Inasmuch as all thymuses shrink with age, thymic hormones—if they existed—could conceivably render service to almost everyone.

This brings us to thymosin, a discovery already mentioned in passing, but perhaps a story worth telling in more detail for at least two good reasons: (1) Thymosin may be one of the first important anti-aging drugs to reach the marketplace; and (2) the story illustrates how research in some other area not officially related to gerontology in any way at the outset can nevertheless make a major contribution to it (in the same way that gerontological research will make major contributions to cancer, genetics, and immunology, which may bypass in importance work done specifically to further knowledge in those fields). By 1966, Allan L. Goldstein, a young biochemist then working at the Albert Einstein Medical College in New York in collaboration with his colleague and mentor, Abraham White, had discovered and isolated the hormone which they named thymosin. White and Goldstein have both now long since left New York, but they have continued to coordinate their efforts. White went to Palo Alto, where he has been dividing his time between Syntex Research and Stanford University. Goldstein meanwhile was invited to become director of the biochemistry division at the University of Texas Medical Branch (UTMB) in Galveston, where he quickly recruited a superb and dedicated team of young, energetic investigators. With a high-priority effort financed in part by the government, in part by foundations, in part by private Texas contributors, and in part by Hoffmann-LaRoche, Goldstein was able to crash ahead with the development of thymosin. Members of the team worked out new immuno-assays and new ways of extracting and purifying the hormone, and they ascertained that thymosin does circulate in the human bloodstream and decreases with age; and, further, that bovine thymosin is sufficiently similar to be active on human cells and can turn immature human stem cells into mature T-lymphocytes. Soon nearly a hundred other laboratories around the world were participating in thymosin research, and it has already begun to be used on human patients.

The first patients to benefit will be those with genetic immune deficiencies. A few of these victims—those born without the capacity to make stem cells at all—may turn out to be beyond the reach of thymosin. For these, bone-marrow transplants, always a tricky and hazardous procedure, may be the only alternative for some time to come. But for the majority of immune-deficient patients, thymosin should be able to help—just as the lymphocyte injections were able to help the dwarf mice—and even to restore them to complete immunological normality.

There are many other areas where thymosin, with its presumed capacity to boost the immune system, may have direct benefits. One is cancer. If Burnet's immunological-surveillance theory is correct, then thymosin may well restore the body's cell-mediated ability to hold off malignancy. Such experiments are already under way at UTMB and elsewhere.

In the same manner, thymosin may hold off the aging process itself. The body's immunity, as we have seen, does decrease with age; so do the quantities of thymosin circulating in the blood—and so does the capacity of the thymus to produce new lymphocytes. New supplies of thymosin added to the circulation should increase resistance to all kinds of infections, to cancer, and to all manner of deteriorative changes, thus enhancing well-being and good health over a much longer period of years. This hypothesis, too, is already being tested in a preliminary way with aging cells in tissue culture, by Goldstein, Walford, and Makinodan, among others.

It is obvious, then, that thymosin is a hopeful therapy for that aspect of immunity which has to do with lowered efficiency, hence less protection, as we age. But what of those instances where the immune system is functioning very actively but against our best interests, as in the case of transplant rejection, or autoimmunity?

When tissue is grafted onto or into our bodies, we would obviously wish those cells to be unmolested, inasmuch as we have transplanted them on purpose, to improve our chances of survival. But those cells are unmistakably foreign, and the immune system—in this case, the T-cells in a direct cell-mediated attack—goes after them with lethal intent. Could thymosin help? Yes, in a way. What we could hope for is the development of an *anti-thymosin serum*.

Under present circumstances, transplant teams use a variety of immunosuppressive techniques, some of them fairly radical, to knock out the T-cell system (and usually the B-cell system as well, since there is no way to suppress them selectively). Anti-thymosin might be a gentler way to knock out the system, and then *only the T-cell system,* leaving the B-cells free to continue making antibodies against the bacterial infections which have killed many patients after an otherwise successful transplant. Moreover, once all the old lymphocytes were wiped out, thymosin could stimulate the production of new, mature lymphocytes from stem cells. These new lymphocytes would not have inherited any of the old memories, hence might very well accept the formerly foreign graft tissue as legitimate if "naturalized" parts of the body; in that case, no rejection would occur.

A similar effect might be achieved in autoimmune diseases. In such a disease, usually (though not invariably) late in life, autoimmunity may come to pass either because aging changes in the attacked cells make them look foreign to our lymphocytes (Makinodan believes this is what happens about 90 per cent of the time) or because aging changes in the lymphocytes themselves have blurred their "judgment." In either case, newly constituted lymphocytes might again accept these changed cells as being part of the self rather than enemies. In autoimmunity, incidentally, this blurred judgment can occur in either B-cells or T-cells—in either the humoral or cell-mediated immune systems. In the case of humoral autoimmunity, the B-cells produce copious quantities of "autoantibodies." In a case like that, what could thymosin possibly do about B-cells and antibodies? This: Under normal circumstances, the T-lymphocytes have an additional function I have so far not mentioned. There exist a class of T-cells known as suppressor lymphocytes, which actually step in and inhibit the B-cells from making too many antibodies. Presumably thymosin, if it could restore the body's T-cell population to normal, could thereby once more keep antibody production in balanced control. Where autoimmunity is cell-mediated, with

T-cells themselves attacking other body cells they mistake as foreign, our hope would reside, as in transplant rejection, with the development of anti-thymosin.

If it turns out, as many now suspect, that rheumatoid arthritis, pernicious anemia, late-onset diabetes, Hashimoto's thyroiditis, systemic lupus erythematosis, and multiple sclerosis, among others, are autoimmune diseases, then thymosin*—if it can defeat autoimmunity —could have a broad impact indeed, not only in delaying senescence but in making the later years considerably more comfortable.

* Most endocrine glands secrete more than one hormone, and the same may be true of the thymus. Thymosin may be only one of a family of hormones. In fact, another Goldstein—Gideon Goldstein, formerly of New York University and now with Sloan-Kettering—is working with other thymic hormones, thymopoietin I and II.

Chapter X

HORMONES AND
ENZYMES

Though thymosin is the most striking example, other hormones have long been known to be involved—either by their presence or by their absence—in the aging process. The rejuvenating effects of certain sex hormones, for instance, administered as replacement therapy when the natural supply has run down, are widely recognized. A pioneering researcher in this area used to be William H. Masters (of Masters and Johnson) before he shifted his focus from the impersonal biology of sex to its more intimate physiological and psychosocial aspects. A presentation he gave at the annual meeting of the American Gynecological Society in 1957 ("Sex Steroid Influences on the Aging Process," later published in the *American Journal of Obstetrics and Gynecology*) was probably the best survey available at that time. (Masters was also interested in thyroid and adrenal hormones in relation to aging.) Naturally, much work has been done since 1957, and the best summarizer of that information —to which his own work has of course contributed—has been USC's Caleb Finch, who is firmly convinced that "the extent of changes in the endocrine system has direct bearing on all theories of aging, as well as on the treatment of diseases in older persons."

Almost every experiment probing for clues to the link between hormones and aging has pointed to centralized endocrine control in the brain—and specifically to the hypothalamus and pituitary, the master-control sites of the entire autonomous (endocrine) nervous system, and apparently the major channels of communication with the central nervous system as well.

Much research has been devoted to the reproductive hormones.

This is a natural area for study, inasmuch as the sexual and procreative functions, especially in females, tend to be cyclical, and the organism arrives at a point in life where such cycles come to an end. Moreover, these cyclical functions are known to be regulated by specific hormones. A likely question for any investigator is: When the ovarian and estrous cycles in aging females come to a halt, does this represent a failure of the reproductive tract itself, or of the central endocrine control systems of the brain?

Seeking a solution, Joseph Meites and his associates at Michigan State University were able repeatedly to reactivate ovulation in female rats (who were well past the age when ovulation could reasonably be expected to occur naturally) by means of electrical brain stimulation and the injection of progesterone, epinephrine, L-dopa, and iproniazid. This clearly pointed to the brain centers as the sites of hormonal "aging" rather than the old ovaries themselves, which, when properly stimulated, were perfectly capable of producing eggs.

When a team at the University of Milan—A. Pecile, E. Müller, and G. Falconi—removed the pituitary from a young adult female rat and replaced it with the pituitary of an old rat, the young ovaries and uterus atrophied prematurely. Following these leads, and arriving at similar results and conclusions, Ming-tsung Peng and Hive-ho Huang of Taipei's National Taiwan University transplanted both ovaries and pituitaries in several variations of the same theme. To clinch the matter, G. B. Talbert and P. L. Krohn in England— transplanting ova rather than whole ovaries—found that, in young females, old eggs could produce the same quantity and quality of normal offspring as young eggs could; whereas, in old females, young eggs were seldom able to produce offspring at all. The only question that remained, in the words of Peng and Huang (reporting their research in *Fertility and Sterility*) was "which part of the hypothalamic-pituitary axis plays the primary role in reproductive dysfunction in old female rats."

The hypothalamic-pituitary axis is of course not the only brain site where hormones are active. An international conference of neuroendocrinologists held in 1974 at the University of North Carolina School of Medicine made it clear that hormones are both active and interactive in many areas of the brain—though the interactions are often poorly understood; but the control centers do seem to reside in that restricted region. Of some interest, incidentally, especially when one considers Denckla's theories, is a presentation given at that conference by Walter E. Stumpf of North Carolina. "Thyroid hormones—or metabolites of them—which are thought to exert relatively little effect on mature brain tissue in contrast to the developing brain," Stumpf (and Lester D. Grant) reported in *Science,* "appeared to be localized in nuclei and cytoplasm of neurons almost throughout the entire mature brain." If thyroid hormones or their products are essential for the function of mature brain cells—which would seem to be the case in the light of this finding—and are present both in the nucleus and cytoplasm of each cell, it certainly makes sense that thyroid deprivation would have a series of deleterious effects on those cells, which could evince themselves as cross-linkages, error catastrophes, lipofuscin accumulations, and other "causes" of aging. But let us return to that idea in the next chapter.

The experiments we were discussing a moment ago dealt almost entirely with the hormones of sex and reproduction, which are quite special and may not be typical of all hormones. But then, no hormones are "typical." Hormone function of any variety is a complicated business. Some hormones seem to have only one function, others have several. Some seem to act alone, others require interaction with further hormones. Some need to be triggered by others and/or may need in turn to trigger yet others before the assigned task can be carried out. How hormones act and react depends a great deal on the environment (which they may help create) in and around the endocrine glands, in the bloodstream which transports them, and in and around the target cells—which possess "hormone receptor sites" that may or may not be receptive at a given moment, or whose receptivity may go up or down (mostly down) with aging.

In order to function successfully in any cell, whether in the nucleus or the cytoplasm, a hormone must set off or "induce" the appropriate enzyme activity. Because enzymes are so specific in their own functions, the study of "enzyme induction" has been a handy way to measure hormonal action—and especially to see how this action is affected by the passage of time. Richard C. Adelman of the Temple University Medical School in Philadelphia, the leading investigator in this area, prefers to call what he measures "enzyme adaptation." It is well known that all mortal organisms adapt with increasing difficulty to environmental stress as they age. In fact they have trouble adapting to any environmental change, because, with approaching senescence, change itself constitutes stress. And since change never stops, stress is fairly constant, until eventually death brings an end—not to change, since change goes on, but to that individual life as a historical entity.

As one of a myriad examples of stress adaptation, Samuel Rosen —the New York ear surgeon famous for inventing the "stapes mobilization" operation that cures one type of deafness—cites the manner in which human organisms adapt to noise. Noise is a form of stress, and we react to it not only with our auditory organs but with our cardiovascular systems as well. Rosen has made many measurements among the inhabitants of many cultures, and has established this relationship beyond doubt. "Whenever we hear a loud noise," he says, "our blood vessels contract. If the noise is continuous, then our vessels keep reacting. A young person's cardiovascular system—and ears—recover much more quickly than those of an older person. If I were to spend three hours in a discotheque with my son, my body would take much longer than his to return to normal."

On a cellular and molecular level, our biochemical adaptations also seem to slow down. Over many years, more than a hundred enzymes were studied and more than a thousand papers published; yet, though some tantalizing hints were turned up, the massive body of data led to no very helpful conclusions. That was the situation when Adelman appeared on the scene. (Around the same time, Finch, too, was contributing some valuable insights—especially a new appreciation of the importance of this type of research.) In the case of one enzyme after another, when challenged with a given hormone, Adelman's careful investigations revealed that in rats aged from two to twenty-four months the *time of reaction*—the time it took the specific cellular enzymes to respond to the hormones—went up in proportion to the animal's age. Even in those cases where the given enzyme activity finally reached the same level in an old rat as in a young one, it took correspondingly longer to reach that level. In order to make the kind of meticulous studies necessary to pinpoint where in the complex chain of hormone action the slowdown occurred, Adelman established a large colony of a specially bred variety of male laboratory rats known as the Sprague-Dawley strain. The rats were allowed to age normally, under protected circumstances, for the main purpose of studying their enzyme adaptation as they grew older. Environmental conditions were kept as constant as possible, even to the extent of providing, throughout their life-times, a pasteurized, sterilized diet whose components were rigidly controlled so that none of the biochemical measurements could be attributed either to microbial infections or to nutritional differences.

With this system, as free of boobytraps as human ingenuity could make it, Adelman proceeded with his studies, using various hormones and measuring the adaptive capacity of many enzymes. His most intensive investigations, however, centered on two hormones—corticosterone and insulin—and two liver enzymes—glucokinase and tyrosine aminotransferase (TAT). Adelman made this decision because it was known that: (1) the adaptive capacity of both these enzymes can deteriorate with age; and (2) the presence of these two hormones stimulates the activity of these enzymes. As an example: if you administer glucose, you get liver glucokinase activity —but only if insulin is present. Adelman found that, with carefully controlled injections of insulin to rats of various ages, there was no loss of glucokinase adaptability with aging. Both in magnitude of activity and speed of response, the twenty-four-month-old rats did as well as the two-month-old rats! (Finch and others got similar results.) Meanwhile Adelman's colleagues and students ascertained, in other painstaking experiments, that the binding of insulin to its receptor molecules in old liver cells was just as efficient as in young liver cells. So the problems in adaptation with aging were *not* in the responses of the cells or in the receptor molecules. Eliminating one possibility after another, Adelman arrived at the conclusion that the slowing of enzyme adaptation with age was due to either the lesser availability, or the lessened effectiveness, of the hormone itself— probably as a result of a deficiency at the hypothalamic-pituitary level.

While these experiments were in progress, other rats were being studied for their TAT activity in response to the adrenal steroid hormone, corticosterone. Under ordinary circumstances, the pituitary first releases the hormone ACTH, which triggers the adrenal glands to secrete corticosterone into the bloodstream. When his rats were injected with ACTH, Adelman found that the old rats had just as much corticosterone circulating in their bloodstreams—and were able to maintain it at the same levels—as the young rats did. So the aging problem wasn't there either. And the liver-cell enzymes were just as responsive to the hormone as was the case with gluco-kinase and insulin. Again, cellular-molecular failure was ruled out, and again the hypothalamic-pituitary axis was implicated, because it seemed only logical that the pituitary must be releasing a lowered supply of ACTH.

A further experiment made the argument even more convincing. As an adaptive mechanism in a stress situation—such as a short period of starvation—higher levels of corticosterone would appear in the bloodstream. Adelman subjected his rats to just such a short period of starvation, and found that in two-month-old rats corticosterone levels went up several fold; at twelve months, the levels went up only slightly; and at twenty-four months of age, there was no response at all. Adelman looked for alternate explanations of these results. Could it be that, to older rats, food was of less importance, and the short period of starvation simply not very stressful? Adelman was soon able to ascertain that this was not the case. Without going through the entire chain of further experimentation and reasoning, he finally concluded, in a 1974 lecture before the annual meeting of the American Association for the Advancement of Science: "We have been able to demonstrate for the first time that a neuroendocrinological lesion of aging, probably localized within or near the hypothalamus, is capable of altering the pattern of liver enzyme adaptation."

Adelman's results are extremely encouraging, for a variety of reasons. One is that, if aging bodies have an unimpaired capacity to maintain normal levels of hormones in their bloodstreams, and if the cells have an unimpaired capacity to receive and use them, then the probability is higher that anti-aging hormones, when administered, will restore cellular functions—which are, after all, not gone but only waiting for the necessary stimulation. This does not, of course, mean that all cell functions can be restored by hormones; though such an idea is not preposterous. (We should exercise caution in extrapolating liver-cell activity to other cells. Liver cells, remember, retain more regenerative powers than other postmitotic cells—e.g., nerve and muscle cells—and it's likely that fewer of their genetic switches are turned off permanently. Dieter Platt and his associates at the University of Giessen School of Medicine in Germany have studied the varying response, with age, of lysosomal enzymes [the lysosome is one of the organelles in the cytoplasm of all cells]. They found that the lysosomal enzymes of the liver were, in general, much more stable than those of the spleen or the brain.)

Another hope which Adelman's work offers is a means for

measuring physiological senescence via the cells' enzyme-adaptive capacities. His insulin studies should give us some important insights into "maturity-onset" diabetes, and his general approach should offer some clues as to why certain liver tumors can be chemically produced in aging organisms, not to mention new tools for determining both the safety and efficacy of a variety of drugs and hormones in elderly patients. Dieter Platt was able to demonstrate, for instance, that lysosomal enzyme activity is quite age-dependent in its response to phenobarbital. A number of other German investigators got similar results with other drugs. These studies are further corroborated by a long series of rat experiments carried out with amphetamines, barbiturates, tranquilizers, anesthetics, and anticonvulsants by Ryuichi Kato and Akira Takanaka at Tokyo's National Institute of Hygienic Sciences.

Virtually all the data from hormone and enzyme studies—though there remain vast gaps in our knowledge—lead Caleb Finch to at least partial agreement with Denckla: that the aging clock is in the brain, that it is located in the hypothalamic-pituitary endocrine-control center, and that whatever is responsible for the aging changes that occur there, they in turn produce a "cascade effect" of changes throughout the organism. There is nothing in this view to contradict Denckla's further contentions, however. His death hormones, if they exist, would be capable of causing aging changes anywhere in the body, including the hypothalamic-pituitary control centers (which thus literally self-destruct). They could turn off the thymus and interfere in other ways with immune functions. V. V. Frolkis, another advocate of the brain-endocrine clock and himself a brilliant and original investigator, has also shown that the same set of mechanisms may well be in control of the cardiovascular system. The immune and cardiovascular, remember, are the two systems whose failure, according to Denckla, is what kills us all. His death hormone, principally by denying the cells their thyroid (and perhaps their thymic) hormones, could theoretically do the whole job.

Still another Soviet researcher, V. M. Dilman of Leningrad's N. N. Petrov Research Institute of Oncology, pinpoints the hypothalamus as the probable suppressor of vital activities whose decline leads to aging and death, and he believes this hypothalamic activity is genetically programmed. But Dilman believes that the hypothalamus—and the pituitary, which it stimulates—does not so much act as *react* to information fed back from the body. When the biochemistry reaches a certain state of readiness for the next stage of the genetic program, it signals the hypothalamus to release its suppressors. Dilman's theory seems in no basic way to contradict Denckla's. If all this is proven to be correct, would a cellular clock of aging then be ruled out? Not at all—for the same reasons stated at the end of the last chapter.

We are ready now for a closer look at some further experiments which may help us move nearer to what I like to think of as a "unified field theory" of aging.

Chapter XI

ACCELERATED AGING
IN NATURE

"May I have the slide? . . . What a splendid creature this salmon is, on its way to spawn!" Next slide: "And look at *this* forlorn hulk—a fish that has lately done so [spawned]. Note the humped back, the hooked jaw, and the fungus mottling its skin. Soon it will be dead and drifting downstream. This is the fate of all five Pacific species of salmon." The speaker was Nobel virologist Peyton Rous, on the occasion of awarding the Kober Medal (of the Association of American Physicians) in 1961 to British-born O. H. Robertson, who elucidated, for the first time, the mechanisms involved in the obscenely swift senescence of the Pacific salmon. This "splendid creature," as seen in Peyton Rous's first slide, freely roams the vast sweeps of the Pacific Ocean for two or three years until, one day, the pre-set biological alarm goes off—the call to spawn, imperious, unrefusable. Swimming day and night, it heads like a torpedo for the coast from which it first came, guided by a fantastic inner navigational ability that no human scientist can yet explain. Driven by the same internal command, it moves upriver (see Chapter I) on an incredible journey to its inland spawning grounds—perhaps the very spawning grounds where it first came to life, almost literally over the dead bodies of its parents. The magnificent condemned fish neither rests nor eats once it hits the fresh water of the river. And as soon as its reproductive function is achieved, it quickly turns into the soft-boned, rotten-fleshed "forlorn hulk" of Slide Two.

Some have speculated that the very coming-in-from-the-sea, the passage from salt water to fresh, somehow triggers the onset of senescence even as the salmon spends its last heroic energies running the obstacle course against gravity to its life-in-death rendezvous. More recent studies than Robertson's have been made in British Columbia by a multinational team of scientists aboard the *Alpha Helix,* the marvelously equipped research vessel of the Scripps Institution of Oceanography. These newer studies have shown that the totally preoccupied fish may quite literally starve to death, denying itself any nutritional refueling of its vanishing energies and at the same time rendering itself unable to produce the mucus that protects the gills which filter its oxygen; so it is deprived of oxygen as well as nutrients.

The change from salt water to fresh *could* be important in some varieties of salmon, inasmuch as such changes in environment do often trigger changes in biological activity, as Stewart Wolf—director of the Marine Biomedical Institute at UTMB/Galveston—points out. As one example, Wolf cites the case of a shark whose liver, under normal circumstances, resembles that of an alcoholic human's, cirrhotic and full of fat. It does not manufacture any protein and contains a high concentration of urea, which would represent advanced kidney failure in a human body. If that shark is moved from its customary salt-water habitat and put into fresh water, the urea levels quickly fall, and the shark's liver begins making albumin!

Nevertheless, O. H. Robertson dismissed the likelihood that the mere change from salt water to fresh could wholly account for the multitudinous, simultaneous biological transformations which he observed taking place. He dismissed the idea because he found a breed of salmon called the kokanee—a dwarf blueback variety—that lived in land-locked lakes. They spent their lives in fresh water and never got out to sea at all; yet they underwent the same rapid degeneration after spawning as the migratory varieties. For this very reason, the kokanee proved to be Robertson's favorite experimental animal; it was simply easier to keep track of throughout its life cycle.

Though Robertson's studies of the salmon probably represent the work for which he will be best remembered, he did not begin this research until after his official retirement from the University of Chicago. During World War I, as part of Harvey Cushing's Harvard Unit in France, Robertson created the first blood bank. At a later stage of his long and varied medical career in many parts of the world, Robertson's investigations had given him some critical insights into the nature of lobar pneumonia; but his findings were never put to use because, just then, antibiotics came along, and his further research seemed no longer necessary. On retiring, Robertson moved back to California, where he had spent a good part of his childhood (his Scottish parents moved there from England when he was two years old), to accept a lectureship at Stanford. From his new home base in the Santa Cruz mountains, he embarked on the salmon experiments, which were often as frustrating as they were painstaking. Once, after he had labored with the assistance of his friend, pediatric surgeon Clifford Sweet, to perform some 200 delicate laparotomies (surgical sections of the abdominal wall) on fingerlings in the Lake Tahoe hatchery, a hungry raccoon came along and devoured most of his experiment. But he persisted, working with several species of salmon, eliminating one possible cause after another—including sheer exhaustion or starvation—as the major explanation of the rapid aging phenomenon.

He eventually ruled out everything except endocrine dysfunction —some sort of drastic hormonal imbalance. And so it turned out to be. Robertson found that, in a process that probably began even before spawning, the salmon's adrenal cortex grew to many times its normal size while, at the same time, the pituitary also enlarged and its control capacities degenerated—resulting in an enormous overproduction of corticosteroids. As Peyton Rous (and Stewart Wolf and Donner Denckla, among others) has noted, this strongly resembles what happens in Cushing's syndrome (the same celebrated Cushing under whom Robertson did his wartime service) in human patients, where a great overbalance of glucocorticoids causes widespread and often severe symptoms. This violent hormonal disturbance could certainly account for the variegated senescent changes that ensue at such an accelerated pace in the salmon. The way Rous characterized the process is prophetic of Denckla: "death control, effected through an intrinsic mechanism"—an intrinsic hormonal mechanism, at that.

Denckla speculates that what happens in Cushing's syndrome and in the senescent Pacific salmon is similar to what may happen in individual human cells. As the organism ages, and the pituitary releases its death hormones, the cell is prevented from taking up thyroxine for its vital metabolic needs. Though the glucocorticoids within the cell do not increase in quantity, they are in sudden oversupply when the thyroid hormone is not there to counterbalance their effects. As a consequence, the cell is afflicted with a kind of

Cushing's syndrome in miniature, which could result in a variety of aging changes, from free radicals and cross-linkages to somatic mutations and error catastrophes. This would occur throughout the body, though the deterioration, subtle at the start (in puberty) and growing more pronounced only with further releases of the "anti-thyroid" hormone later in life, would proceed at a statelier pace than in the salmon.

Not that the salmon story can be considered as all told. Other scientists continue to study the Pacific varieties in more systematic ways than were available to Robertson. Among them are Andrew A. Benson and Walter Garey of the Scripps Institution in La Jolla, California, who were the leaders of the *Alpha Helix* expedition. The vessel's pioneering salmon-study voyage, which lasted through many months of 1968 and included some side projects at remote inland sites in British Columbia, was made by a team of thirty-seven scientists from Canada, the United States, Israel, and France. Igor Lobanov Rostovsky has written a beautiful account of the whole expedition, evoking its continuing sense of physical and intellectual adventure, in a magazine called *Oceans*.

"Not many of the men," writes Rostovsky, "had ever seen salmon except in a can or a fish market. Specialists in metabolism and human disorders (including ten doctors of medicine), their collective expertise encompassed: bone disease, milk protein, intestinal pathology (specializing in children), cell ultrastructure, brain diseases, glandular disorders, atherosclerosis and cardiovascular diseases." They studied four varieties of salmon: pink, chub, coho, and sockeye.

Their findings have already shed a great deal of new light on the tragically accelerated events that highlight the last days of the salmon—findings that should lead to many human applications. For instance, Don Puppione of the Donner Laboratory of Medical Physics in Berkeley was astounded to discover that, just before spawning, the salmon's bloodstream contained twenty times the amount of fatty compounds—including cholesterol—found in normal human blood; yet none of it seems to accumulate in the arteries! "From the salmon," says Puppione, "we may learn how to make a serum of lipoprotein that will not settle out in the human aorta. If we can find out how the fish holds his fat and protein together in serum lipoprotein, then perhaps we can learn how to feed a human being so that he makes this type of fat carrier in his blood."

Meanwhile Douglas Copp of the University of British Columbia School of Medicine was studying a tiny gland no bigger than a grain of rice. (The hormone it produces, incidentally, may prove useful in human bone and metabolic disorders.) "Situated behind the gills and in front of the heart," writes Rostovsky, "this minuscule, secreting organ is actually the *embryological precursor of the thyroid gland in humans*. Dr. Copp found that *this gland vanishes after the fish spawns*." (The italic emphasis is mine.) This would seem to score another point for Denckla: the pituitary goes out of control and overproduces, while the thyroid component disappears.

In the salmon we seem to have occurring simultaneously the two diseases—both of them endocrine disorders—that most mimic aging in human patients: hypothyroidism (too little thyroid hormone) and hyperadrenocorticism (too much of the adrenal hormones, the corticosteroids, as in Cushing's syndrome). And they are without much doubt genetically programmed. As Rostovsky points out, "during a fortnight . . . the pink salmon's physiology runs through the steps of deterioration that may extend from 20 to 40 years in the life of a human being." Thus it makes an ideal model for gerontological study.

It was Eberhard G. Trams of the National Institute of Neurological Diseases and Stroke who especially concentrated on the brain and hormonal aspects of the salmon's senescence (and has continued to do so). He noted, as Robertson did but in more precise detail, the enlarged pituitary (three times as big in fresh water as in the ocean), the steroid overproduction, and other physiological changes. He also observed that the salmon died of "a complete metabolic shutdown," and that the increased production of adrenal steroids seemed to *inhibit antibodies,* thereby leaving the fish more vulnerable to infection: score points for Walford and Burnet, but also for Denckla again.

On the whole, the recent findings substantiate Robertson's in terms of hormonal causation, but it is now clearer that the process is already taking place during the entire time the salmon is journeying upriver. It could be that whatever impels the fish to undertake its amazing trip is the same trigger that sets in motion the decay processes—the compulsive behavior leading to the starvation leading to the glandular malfunctions in falling domino fashion.

But perhaps not. Hear, for instance, one more fish story—the steelhead trout's. The steelhead trout, like the salmon, comes in from the ocean and swims upriver to its spawning grounds, and also undergoes rapid degeneration. But Robert Van Citters of the University of Washington in Seattle discovered, some years ago, that the steelhead trout *do not all die*. Moreover, those that do survive and reach the ocean once more are somehow regenerated and rejuvenated! The terrible—presumably lethal—arterial lesions simply disappear. Using radioactive tracers, Van Citters ascertained that some of the trout were able to spawn, degenerate, and regenerate at least two or three times, apparently with no permanent damage. Rediscovering Van Citters's neglected work, Stewart Wolf is eager to do followup studies of the mechanisms that permit the trout's remarkable recovery. Can the trout teach us something about reversing human degenerative processes? Wolf is seeking support for the building of an artificial trout stream at or near UTMB's Galveston campus in order to pursue these investigations.

If the Pacific salmon and the steelhead trout represent nature's experiments—perhaps inadvertent—in accelerated aging processes, there is a fortunately rare human disease which serves as a similar gerontological model for similar reasons. The disease is progeria— also known as the Hutchinson-Gilford syndrome, after the two British doctors who independently described it in the late nineteenth century—which the *Journal of the American Medical Association* once headlined as "Nature's Experiment in Unnatural Aging." According to Franklin L. DeBusk of the University of Florida, who undertook an exhaustive survey of the literature (reported in *Journal of Pediatrics*), progeria occurs no more than once in 8 million births, and he was able to find reports of only sixty cases of progeria, worldwide, as of April 1972.

There cannot be too many childhood diseases that are more tragic. The progeria victim appears, for a period of anywhere from six months to three years, to be perfectly normal in every respect—just as his height and weight were normal at birth. But then disquieting signs begin to appear. Growth is retarded, and the progeric child, if he survives through his teens, never gets to be any bigger than a normal three- to five-year-old. As soon as his telescoped childhood is over, other changes begin to take place. These have been described in several papers in the *Journal of the American Geriatrics Society* by William Reichel, director of the Family Medicine and Human

Development Program at the Franklin Square Hospital in Baltimore, who has made the study of progeria (and the similar, later-appearing disease, Werner's syndrome) his lifelong avocation.

The typical progeric child begins to look frail and old as early as the age of three or four. He may start experiencing cardiac troubles as early as five, though often not until ten or fifteen, and these troubles may include heart murmurs, atherosclerosis, elevated cholesterol levels, high blood pressure, angina pectoris, congestive heart failure—and finally the heart attack that is the most usual cause of death. The average life span of progerics is twelve to eighteen years, though some have died as early as five (DeBusk believes those who died between five and seven were really the victims of accidents, and that seven is the earliest death from "old age"), and some have survived to the age of twenty-seven. For the most part, though, it is an early-teen-age death, after a long period of steady and irreversible debilitation and deterioration. The progeric is a dwarf, but with a head that is of normal size and therefore looks larger than normal compared to the stunted body. The skin is wrinkled and parchment-like, also almost opaque, with virtually no fat under the skin and the blood vessels showing prominently. The hair is gray and sparse—if any remains at all. The face is birdlike, the eyes protuberant, the nose hooked. In fact, progeria patients, as DeBusk points out, "bear an uncanny resemblance to one another." They are weak-limbed and stiff-jointed, and no medication or therapy has yet been found that will help them.

What perhaps renders their plight even more tragic, Reichel suggests, is the fact that they retain normal intelligence, hence are sensitive to the implications of their condition. "These children," DeBusk observes, "tended to be shy and aware of their unusual appearance. They were friendly, lively, witty and mischievous in the company of acquaintances, and they exhibited normal emotions, becoming happy, angry, and sad in the appropriate situations." Harvard's Dorothy B. Villee adds, in *Pediatrics,* that "their major complaint is the social problems produced by the stigma of their appearance."

Though progeria undoubtedly *mimics* old age, its victims do not show all the signs of senescence (senile dementia is absent, for example), hence there are reservations about looking upon what happens as true aging. The similarities in symptoms could be sheer coincidence. Reichel asks: "Is it truly a disease of accelerated aging? Does it in fact represent a genetic error? If so, is there one genetic mechanism regulating man's normal life span? Or conversely: Is there a gene or group of genes whose purpose is to facilitate the incorporation of errors into a biological system? If so, does progeria represent an early activation of such a mechanism?" The questions must remain, for the moment, rhetorical.

Progeric children do not seem to have any gross chromosomal abnormalities. Though various studies have cast suspicion on the hormonal and immunological abnormalities of some progerics, the findings have not been consistent, and there exists no conclusive evidence that it is basically either a hormonal or an immunological disease. Reichel has found large accumulations of lipofuscin—the "aging pigment"—in the cells of progerics, as well as abnormalities in the connective tissue. As already mentioned, Samuel Goldstein of McMaster was able to coax only a few divisions out of progeric cells *in vitro*. Betty Shannon Danes of the New York Hospital–Cornell Medical Center has also reported, in *The Journal of Clinical Investigation*, that progeric cells have a lowered cloning efficiency, as well as a diminished capacity to duplicate their DNA or to divide normally (all those deficiencies logically go together, of course). And a Harvard team has turned up suggestive evidence of faulty DNA-repair mechanisms in progeric cells.

No one group of people seems to be singled out as progeria victims. The cases are spread over many nations, and the disease seems to afflict blacks as readily as whites, males as readily as females. There are only three reports of more than one victim in a single family, and only one case that might have resulted from a consanguineous marriage. Thus, though progeria is suspected of being a genetic disease, much about it remains puzzling, and it has certainly not yet been *proven* to be hereditary in origin.

There is a similar disease, however, which is known to be genetic —Werner's syndrome. Its onset does not occur until somewhere between fifteen and twenty years of age, when most progeria victims are already dead. Some believe Werner's syndrome may be merely a later expression of progeria, as evidenced by some of the other names it goes by: *progeria adultorum, progéria à début tardif.*

The Werner's victim also suffers from arrested growth, though of course not to the same extent as progerics. They are simply much shorter than average in stature, and they too become prematurely gray and bald. (Some of their otherwise normal relatives also turn prematurely gray.) They are prone to the earlier-than-usual arrival of diseases ordinarily associated with aging, such as diabetes mellitus, atherosclerosis, heart disease, and cancer—especially cancer of the connective tissue. They die of what looks like old age in their forties and fifties. Though Werner's syndrome is also rare, it occurs about twice as frequently as progeria.

What are we to glean from diseases such as these?

For one thing, whether we define them as "true" aging or not, there is no doubt that, in both diseases, widespread degenerative changes do take place at the level of both the individual cell and the total organism. Whatever it is that occurs brings on degenerative changes much sooner than would happen in the normal course of events, suggesting strongly that the occurrences are not due to simple wear and tear. The probability appears high that some internal timing mechanism is at work, whether it is identical to the clock of aging or not, and that it affects the entire organism; and, further, that the mechanism is somehow built into the individual's genetic information—perhaps as something added, perhaps as something missing, but in any event as something gone wrong. And the something wrong would seem to be in whatever mechanism regulates the onset and *rate* of deterioration. The defect could be in the molecular-genetic apparatus of the individual cell, passed on to all the body's cells by the original fertilized egg. Or it could be in the hypothalamic-pituitary controls of the endocrine system which affect all cells.

In progeria, it is quite clear very early in life that something has gone radically wrong with the child's development. In Werner's syndrome, it is equally clear that the something-wrong has been postponed (if you compare it with progeria) *on program.* There are other devastating diseases, such as Huntington's chorea, which are genetically triggered late in life; but in the case of Werner's, what is triggered is a whole cascade of degenerative agelike changes. If these can be triggered genetically in Werner's victims, they can be triggered in "normal" individuals at more advanced ages—giving added credence to all genetic-clock theories of aging. The hope in these diseases, as in true aging (which is also, in that case, a genetic disease), is that if a program can be accelerated by accident, it can be slowed down—or reversed—on purpose.

A final note before we leave the salmon: the U.S.S.R.'s V. N. Nikitin, long interested in what happens to DNA and its associated problems with aging, has expressed a special fascination with some salmon experiments carried out separately by his Soviet colleagues G. D. Berdyshev and B. F. Vanyushin in the late 1960's. Before spawning and "premature death," as Nikitin calls it, the quantity of a nitrogenous base known as 5-MC (for 5-methyl-cytosine) in the salmon's DNA goes down considerably, perhaps by as much as half. This, by a chain of bio-logic reasoning, led Vanyushin to suspect "some previously nonfunctioning areas on the DNA molecule that may to some extent act as 'lethal genes' "—in a word, the programmed switching on of an aging-and-death mechanism.

Chapter XII

DECELERATED AGING
IN THE LAB

Now that we have looked at a few of nature's experiments in accelerated aging, it is time to examine a few human-designed experiments which have succeeded in *de*celerating the rate of aging—and, in some cases, perhaps, extending the life span of laboratory animals—by means of (1) lowering temperature, (2) restricting dietary intake, and (3) parabiosis.

It has been known since at least 1917 that reducing body temperature slows the aging process, at least in cold-blooded animals. That year Jacques Loeb and John H. Northrop at the Rockefeller Institute discovered, in a series of now-classic experiments, that they could significantly increase the life spans of fruit flies by keeping them at 19°C instead of the usual 25°C. Other researchers were quick to pursue and confirm their findings. More recently Charles H. Barrows, Jr., of GRC/Baltimore succeeded in doubling the life span of the rotifer—a pond-dwelling creature tinier than the period at the end of this sentence, but nevertheless a multicellular invertebrate organism—by lowering its water temperature from 35°C to 25°C. Others have achieved similar results in fish. Roy Walford, for example, working with his UCLA colleague R. K. Liu, doubled the life span of the South American annual fish, *Cynolebias belottii,* by making the water 5°C or 6°C colder. Moreover, because they found a higher ratio of soluble to insoluble collagen in the colder fish than in controls of the same age, they counted this as a further sign of retarded aging.

"In some cold-blooded animals," says Bernard Strehler, who has done temperature-aging studies of his own, "a tenfold increase in longevity has been achieved by lowering body temperature, without affecting body function." So-called cold-blooded creatures or *poikilotherms* are—unlike warm-blooded animals (*homeotherms*)—presumed to be unable to regulate their own temperatures internally, thus fluctuate with the temperature of their environments; but, as Walford has pointed out, this is not strictly true, since many creatures in this category, especially amphibians and reptiles, can exercise a fair degree of temperature regulation under certain circumstances. Nevertheless, they are certainly more susceptible to influence by their surrounding temperatures. Even in warm-blooded animals, however, the aging rate seems to be slowed by cooling. Recently, Robert Meyers of Purdue cooled monkeys a few degrees by direct manipulation of the "thermostat" in the hypothalamus and thereby increased their life spans. At Michigan State University, Barnett Rosenberg and Gabor Kemeny have been able to achieve similar results by using a drug that turns down the thermostat a few degrees in rats.

"There are no exceptions that I know of to the rule that animals live longer at lower temperatures," says Strehler, in a *Medical World News* interview. "The question is whether long-lived people have slightly lower-than-average body temperatures, because if you apply the same mathematical rule that applies to all the animal studies so far, then a few degrees Centigrade drop in body temperature could add something like 15 to 25 years to human life. And that could account for practically all the difference that one sees in human life span. This requires some study—it might be a good predictive index of longevity."

A number of scientists are now suggesting what science fiction writers have been putting into their plots for a long time—that human life might be extended if people could be taught to hibernate, or put artificially into states of hibernation, like the astronauts in *2001: A Space Odyssey*.* To *hibernate* means literally to pass the winter in a state of sleeplike torpor, though it is used loosely to refer to any state of seasonal or periodic torpor. The bear is the best-known popular example of a hibernator. But some creatures *estivate,* that is, they "hibernate" during the summer instead. Others, such as the hummingbird, go into a state of torpor every night in order

---

* The cryonics movement, to be discussed in a later chapter, advocates freezing (rather than burial or cremation) at death, against the day when future science can thaw and revive those now defined as "dead."

to get through their days. Animals can be tricked by various means into hibernating more than they normally would. "Among hibernating animals," Strehler observes, "those that are forced to hibernate more often tend to live longer." Walford emphasizes the opposite— natural hibernators that are prevented from hibernating live a consequently shortened life span.

Now, what gerontologists aim for is not a life span lengthened only by virtue of periods of hibernation, without adding anything to the *waking* years of life. They do not seek to emulate Rip Van Winkle, who lasted a long time chronologically but whose conscious lifetime did not exceed that of other people. Such people would be like Hayflick's deep-frozen WI-38 cells which, when thawed, "remember" where they are; though they "live longer" chronologically, they go through the same number of doublings. What gerontologists seek in hibernation is some clue that would enable them to slow down the rate of aging—during sleep, during the waking hours, or both—in a way that would add a significant quantity of wideawake, conscious, fully appreciated *living* time to life. Liu and Walford have tried to achieve this sort of feat in rats, so far with only limited success, by using such compounds as the tranquilizer chlorpromazine and marijuana derivatives.

Most people—including many gerontologists—mistakenly believe that cooling automatically produces a lowered metabolic rate. But as Liu and Walford write, in *Gerontologia,* "to assume that lowering body temperature leads to a reduced metabolic rate is incorrect. The two do not necessarily go hand in hand, and the effect of temperature on lifespan cannot be explained in this simple fashion. . . . The metabolic rate is not necessarily decreased, and may in fact be increased. Certain metabolic pathways may be enhanced, others depressed." A great deal of confusion exists about the relationship between metabolic rate, temperature, and aging, and we will return to that topic shortly. But let one example suffice: The African lungfish *Protopterus aethiopicus* can, during estivation, lower its metabolic rate to 15 per cent of normal without lowering its temperature at all. Under extreme drought conditions, the lungfish can remain in this suspended state for two years at a stretch, self-encased in hardened mud. Some years ago, Henry Swan—a former cardiovascular surgeon now at Colorado State University, who first became interested in the phenomenon as a pioneer in the use of hypothermia in open-heart surgery and blood-vessel grafting—imported some lungfish from Uganda, extracted and isolated a substance he called antabalone, and injected it into some white rats. He thus induced a 40 per cent reduction in their metabolic rate while lowering their temperature hardly at all.*

To take advantage of the life-lengthening effects of low temperature, some gerontologists have seriously suggested that people might one day sleep in cooled bedrooms or in slightly chilled waterbeds. But, while the principle of intermittent cooling is valid, these specific techniques would be of dubious benefit. Walford believes a cold environment without an actual lowering of body temperature would offer no advantage. In fact, animals frequently respond to cold exposure by *increasing* their metabolic rate as a compensatory measure. Lowering the environmental temperature might make a difference in the case of poikilotherms, but as Denckla points out, in warm-blooded homeotherms such as ourselves, any effective temperature lowering would have to be at the hypothalamic level— as was achieved by Meyers via direct manipulation and by Rosenberg and Kemeny via the drug route. Certainly more such drugs will be discovered, and this is the direction Strehler feels may be the most promising; but only as an interim measure, of course, while waiting to decipher the genetic on-off switching devices. He warns, however, that "there is no way to predict the long-term side effects of artificially reduced temperature." Some scientists are so concerned about this prospect that they oppose any such experimentation at all. Clarence L. Hebert of NIH, for one, believes it would be most unwise to reduce body temperature artificially, even by two or three degrees, unless the individual were either sedated or anesthetized. He predicts that the subject would feel chilly and uncomfortable, and would do a lot of shivering. Metabolism would, as a result, be sluggish, and so would intellectual processes. To keep someone's temperature thus lowered year in and year out would, in Hebert's opinion, result in earlier death rather than longer life. But in the view of Walford and Liu, the "induction of mild, chronic or intermittent hypothermia in the more thermostable homeotherms, such

---

* Swan offers the terms *metabolic torpor* or *torpidation* to cover all forms of hibernation and estivation, including the daily "hibernation" of creatures like the bat and hummingbird. His lungfish studies drew him into total immersion in these phenomena, virtually a whole new career, resulting in his monumental *Thermoregulation and Bioenergetics: Patterns for Vertebrate Survival*.

as man or the mouse, might significantly prolong lifespan without unfavorably influencing other functions." After surveying the literature, they conclude, "In the temperature range of mild hypothermia, bodily functions may not be depressed to any significant extent. On the whole, pronounced inhibition of metabolic processes are not observed until below 25°C." Meyers's experiments with monkeys do not seem to bear out Hebert's fears—at least not in the short run. And Kemeny and Rosenberg have so far been able to reduce rat temperatures chemically with no obvious adverse effects. They plan to carry out long-term experiments, as do Walford and Liu, and they all seem to agree with Strehler that slight reductions in temperature could probably be well tolerated over a 100-year lifetime.

There is a final feature of these temperature-lowering experiments that is worth special emphasis: Though cooling does seem to extend the life span, it does so only in the *later* stages of life. For instance, in the early investigations of *Drosophila* by Loeb and Northrop, cooling the larva had little effect on the rate of its aging (or, if you prefer, its development), while cooling the insect during its mature imago state did slow its rate of aging. John Maynard Smith of Sussex demonstrated the phenomenon even more elegantly at a later date. He kept one group of fruit flies at 26°C for the first half of their lives, then at 20°C for the last half. With another group he reversed the process, going from cool to hot. What he found was that the first half of life, the developing period, was independent of temperature, while the second half, the maturing and aging period, was quite dependent on temperature—and its rate could be considerably stretched out by cooling. Liu and Walford did a similar experiment, but with an added twist, on their favorite tropical fish, *Cynolebias*. They kept careful track of four groups of fish. The first group spent their lives in water at 20°C. The second remained at 15°C. The third group started out at 15° but later were transferred to 20°. The fourth started out at 20° and were later moved to 15°. As might be expected, the shortest-lived fish were those which spent their whole lives in the warm water, and next in line were those who had moved from cooler to warmer water. But there was one big surprise: the fish who lived longest of all were not those who had spent their lives in cool water but those who had started in warm water and only later moved to cool. Thus Liu and Walford ascertained to their satisfaction that starting out life—in the developing stage—at a warm temperature enabled the fish to derive even greater benefit from the reduced temperatures during their period of maturity and senescence.

Barrows, too, working with his rotifers, found that cooling extended only the latter end of life. But he was eager to follow up another technique for life extension that Northrop had tried at Rockefeller with *Drosophila:* Northrop, experimenting with the effects of food restriction, discovered that periods of *starvation* produced exactly the reverse result of cooling, that is, it stretched out the life span in the early, developmental, larval stages, while the same dietary deprivation had no such effect on the mature imago! The species of rotifer Barrows worked with had a normal life span of about eighteen days. His cooling techniques added an additional eighteen days. When he reduced the food supply by half, Barrows found he could add yet another eighteen days—this time to the early part of the rotifer's life. By combining temperature with diet control, then, he was able to *triple* the life span, adding another whole lifetime, as it were, at each end of life.

It was Clive M. McCay of Cornell who, perhaps taking his cue from Northrop, began to experiment with underfeeding as a means of extending the life spans of rats. McCay's work—which he began in the late 1920's—has also become classic, though it made its impact only slowly. One of McCay's initial motivations was to study the relationship of growth to aging. Some long-lived animals, such as the Galapagos tortoise and certain species of fish, grow slowly and continue to grow throughout their lives. McCay wondered if the pattern of aging in mammals might somehow be related to the fact that life begins with a rapid spurt of growth, then stops altogether when the organism is . . . well, full-grown. McCay started with two groups of very young rats. One group was fed a normal, well-balanced laboratory diet. The other group was also fed a balanced diet, with all the necessary vitamins and minerals, but their caloric intake was drastically reduced to virtually a semi-starvation level (about one-third of normal), in order to slow their growth. McCay did indeed retard their growth and development; in some cases the control rats were senile by the time the underfed rats had reached maturity, their coats still glossy and youthful-looking. On the average, McCay had come close to doubling the life spans of these rats. Of those on the normal diet, the Methuselah of the batch lived only 969 days, while one of the underfed lived as long as 1,465 days. The retarded growth of the calorie-restricted rats did not keep them from being normally active and intelligent; and many were capable of resuming normal growth at a later stage.

"McCay's 1,000-day-old retarded rats," wrote Robert Prehoda in *Extended Youth,* "might be compared to a 90-year-old human with the physical appearance of a teen-ager. . . . McCay disproved the theory that the life-span is species-limited. Of even greater significance, he proved that the mammalian life-span can be doubled and the period of youth as a percentage of the total life-span increased. Every responsible theory of aging must include an explanation of why McCay's retardation experiments were successful."

As an aside, the discovery that underfeeding can prolong life made some investigators skeptical of Denham Harman's results when he began reporting similar results through the administration of antioxidants. Because the antioxidants he used were known to lower the appetite, it was suspected that the longer lives of his mice might be due simply to the fact that they were eating less! Comfort and others went on to confirm Harman's results, as we now know; yet although Harman undoubtedly enabled his animals to live longer than they otherwise would have, it appears to have been the life expectancy that he increased rather than the maximum life span. But that is an already-told story.

McCay's results have now been duplicated in mice, rats, and other species by many scientists around the world—among them Comfort, Strehler, Walford, Denckla, and Nikitin. Probably the most sophisticated veteran investigator in this vein is Morris H. Ross of the Institute for Cancer Research in Philadelphia. One important truth to emerge from these experiments is that mammals—like fruit flies and rotifers—can have their lives prolonged by calorie restriction *only if it is begun very early in life;* not before weaning, of course; nor so early that it would result in damaging malnutrition; but certainly well before puberty. And the diet, though "restricted," cannot be impoverished nutritionally but only calorically. The life expectancy is influenced not merely by quantity but by composition as well. Ross emphasizes the importance of the specific proportions of protein and carbohydrate in these restricted diets. Apart from the anti-aging benefits that result, and the slower growth, there is a considerably reduced incidence of tumors. "Rapid growth rates, structural or biochemical," says Ross, in *Medical World News,* "are not commensurate with prolonged life span and reduced risk of age-associated diseases."

Would calorie restriction have the same effect on people? In a series of studies of long-lived people in regions of Asia, South America, and the Soviet Union made by Harvard's Alexander Leaf—reported in *Hospital Practice* and the *National Geographic,* and later, at greater length, in his book *Youth in Old Age*—there were only a few consistent features in the lives of these people. They were all relatively penurious and hardworking, and all ate a frugal diet—though the content varied—throughout their lives. In that case, one might ask, how come poor people everywhere do not live longer than others? Because they are *too* poor, and their diets lack vital nutritional ingredients. Though the populations studied by Leaf were far from affluent, neither were they poverty-stricken to the point where they could not eat a *proper* diet. They were neither mal-nourished nor undernourished. It's just that they were not sufficiently affluent to be able to afford to *over*eat. There are many stories of isolated tribes, such as the Mabaan of the Sudan, studied by ear surgeon Samuel Rosen, who were practically free of deafness or cardiovascular disease at very advanced ages; but who, when they moved into Khartoum and began to share the diet and stress of city life, also began to acquire all the degenerative ailments of their new fellow citizens. And there are the instructive tales of wartime, such as the experience of those Scandinavian countries occupied by the Germans in World War II. Deprived of their usual high-calorie, high-fat diet, the death rate from heart attack in these populations went down sharply. When "good times" returned and they could resume their former eating habits, the heart-attack death rate also went back up to normal.

Nevertheless, it would be dangerous indeed to try McCay-style experiments on human beings until a great deal more is known about what happens and why. For one thing, gerontologists have little interest in merely prolonging the years of childhood and adolescence (though that might be interesting to study); what they want is an increase of the mature, vigorous years. To eat lightly but nutritiously, however, is probably good advice at any age, barring some special individual circumstances.

* By the time this book appears, Sula Benet's *How to Live to Be 100: The Life Style of the People of the Caucasus* will also have been published.

There seem to be great similarities between the anti-aging effects of cooling and calorie restriction. In both cases, the rate of aging slows down. But the results are not necessarily equivalent in other respects. For instance, while McCay's underfed rats, though they lived longer, were also undersized, Walford's cooled-down fish grew to larger than normal size. This difference could reflect merely the fact that some poikilotherms, such as carp and tortoises, *do* keep on growing as long as they live, while homeotherms, such as rats and mice, do not. Thus, the *Cynolebias,* with more growing time, might be expected to end up bigger. The fish, after all, remain on their normal diets, whereas the rats may be getting so little food that they simply do not have the *substance* required to build the necessary tissue for added growth. This despite the fact—as observed by V. M. Dilman of Leningrad—that during periods of starvation, the production of growth hormone is increased in order to permit the organism to mobilize the fatty acids and convert them into usable energy.

Walford found that underfeeding and cooling both resulted in a definite suppression of the immune system, which seems to confirm that aging and immunity are indeed somehow related. But there is a built-in paradox here, because, in spite of the lowered immune response, these animals are more resistant to infection than control animals, they get fewer tumors, and they reject transplanted tissue less readily. This is the opposite of what one might expect of a lowered immune response. These phenomena will obviously provide us with new insights into the nature of our immune systems.

Prehoda believes—or did believe, in 1968, when he wrote *Extended Youth*—that Bjorksten's cross-linkage theory provides the best explanation of McCay's results. The underfed rats "had so little caloric food that it was quickly metabolized, with fewer cross-linking agents produced as intermediate products in food metabolism." But he also uses the same explanation to account for the immortality of Alexis Carrel's tissue cultures: "There is an almost total absence of cross-linking agents in the nutrient used to maintain tissue cultures." Now that Hayflick has proved that Carrel's cultures were not immortal after all, explanations must be sought elsewhere. This is not to fault Prehoda's logic. At the time, just about everybody believed that Carrel's cultures *were* immortal. I am sure that some of the findings I describe here with reasonably high confidence will also turn out to be not so after all. In science, we can only work with the data that seems most reliable at a given moment.

For a long time, biomedical scientists believed that almost any slowdown in the rate of any of life's processes was accompanied by a slowdown in the metabolic rate. At least as far back as Max Rubner's publications in Germany early in this century, and those of his teacher, T. K. Van Voit, before him—or even back to V. Regnault in France in 1849—it has been axiomatic that the life span is inversely proportional to the metabolic rate. And so it is, on a species basis. The shrew, with a high burning rate, dies in a year or two, while the Galapagos tortoise, with a very slow burn, goes on for a century or two. The hummingbird also has a very high metabolic rate, but it keeps itself going for ten or twelve years by "hibernating" every night—slowing its motor down to a slow idle, as it were. Bats have to do that for twenty hours of the day.

But this does not hold for individuals within a species. We have already heard Walford assure us that cooling does not necessarily produce a lowered metabolic rate. And Denckla, who has carefully reproduced McCay's experiments as well as other variations of the same theme, has ascertained beyond a reasonable doubt that in underfed rats whose growth is retarded, the metabolic rate is higher than in control animals of the same chronological age. Where individuals within a species are concerned, Denckla is convinced, and altogether convincing, on this point: we should abandon the notion that a higher metabolic rate symbolizes a faster burning up of that individual's living time. In experimental cooling or underfeeding, a higher metabolic rate may in fact be necessary to maintain the heat and energy the organism requires to compensate for lowered temperature and food supply. In many mammalian species, the metabolic rate goes *down* with aging. The same is true in human diseases that mimic aging, such as hypothyroidism. In such cases, previously held ideas would logically lead us to expect a rapidly rising metabolic rate to accompany accelerated aging processes. But the opposite is true. If as Denckla hopes, we do discover or synthesize hormones which successfully *un*block the cells' ability to take up thyroxine— thus slowing, halting, or reversing the aging process—he fears that the beneficiaries may become uncomfortably warm as their metabolic rates rise. Presumably ways will be devised, by then, to counteract this side effect. The temperature-lowering drug of Rosenberg and Kemeny might be a possibility, though Denckla doubts that it would work. Perhaps, as an interim measure, some sort of artificial cooling device, like the astronauts' air-conditioned space suits, would be necessary; though a simpler solution is likely.

In the case of McCay's starved rats, their metabolic rates remain higher, at every stage, than control rats of the same chronological age. In Denckla's view, the retardation of the rats' development through underfeeding simply delays the arrival of puberty, thus also delaying the triggering of death-hormone release by the hypothalamus and pituitary. This delay permits the metabolic rate to remain higher than in the unretarded controls, where thyroid blocking is already under way. Denckla's explanation also fits nicely with that of V. M. Dilman, who postulated that the hypothalamus is triggered into activity via signals fed back from the body when it reaches a given stage; when the periods between those stages are lengthened, hypothalamic triggering is to that extent postponed. Among those who believe that the aging program and the early developmental program of life are probably part of a single program clocked by the hypothalamic-pituitary neuroendocrine system is Paola S. Timiras of the University of California at Berkeley. And she suspects—through a number of brain studies—that increasing quantities of serotonin, one of the major neurotransmitters, as the organism ages may have something to do with the feedback-triggering activity Dilman speaks of. Experiments performed in Timiras's lab by Paul E. Segall suggest that she may be right. Segall has been doing dietary-restriction experiments in the style of McCay and his followers—except that Segall has been focusing on a single element of the diet, the essential amino acid called tryptophan. He has found that tryptophan deprivation alone will often retard aging in some of the same ways as McCay's complete calorie-restriction diet. Because tryptophan is a precursor of serotonin biochemically, Segall and Timiras suspected that withholding tryptophan might also slow the production of serotonin; and so it turned out. It is possible, then, that the buildup of serotonin to a certain critical level is what triggers the hypothalamus to action. And if one can delay the critical serotonin buildup, then one can "stop the clock."

Suppose the hormonal triggers Dilman speaks of, perhaps induced by serotonin as Segall and Timiras suggest, lie in those genetic on-off switches in the DNA of a relatively few brain cells—those ones that signal the hypothalamus to send out the "releasing factors" which in turn signal the pituitary to release the appropriate hormones. In that case, if those switches are subject to a strictly timed genetic program, how can they be influenced by outside factors, such as the restriction of calories? Why do they not turn on, no matter what, at the pre-programmed moment? The probability is that such a genetic program would not be set according to the strict passage of *time* as measured by the mechanical clocks we have devised to coincide with the earth's movements around the sun, but rather according to the stages of the organism's own physiological *development*. These stages are timed events, to be sure, but the timing is sequential rather than absolute. One would expect, then, that if a given stage of development can be artificially delayed, the signal that usually goes back to those critical brain cells to indicate the organism's readiness for the next stage would also be delayed.

But before we come back to some key insights into the nature of genetic switching, let us consider the results of just one more experimental technique, parabiosis. In parabiosis, an aging rat is hooked up to a young rat of the same carefully bred species so that they share a common blood circulation, like Siamese twins. They are joined tail-to-shoulder, which leaves them fairly free to move around. For the aging rat, parabiosis acts as a youth transfusion. In studies with more than 500 parabiotic rats, Frederic C. Ludwig of the University of California at Irvine has found that his older subjects live significantly beyond their expected life span. Something in the blood of the younger rats enabled the older rats to live long after all their unhooked-up littermates were dead. "When rats are joined parabiotically," says Zdanek Hruza of New York University, "remarkable biochemical changes take place." The older rats' cholesterol levels, for instance, go down "almost miraculously."

Several years earlier, at GRC/Baltimore, Dietrich Bodenstein used parabiosis to create Siamese-twin cockroaches—again, young joined to old. Young cockroaches can regenerate lost limbs, but old roaches lose this capacity. In parabiotic union, however, the old roach recovered its regenerative powers. When Bodenstein lopped off a limb, it was promptly regrown. This renewal was attributed to the transference of juvenile hormone from the young roach to its Siamese twin. Could something similar be happening to the rats? Hruza originally suspected the phenomenon to be hormonal in nature but finally concluded that, if a hormone is involved, it cannot be any of the known hormones. What, then, is the nature of the "youth factor" which appears to circulate in the blood of a young rat and transfers its longevous benefits to the senior partner? Could this factor be isolated and used to prolong life without the need for a troublesome parabiotic connection? And could the same be done for people?

It is possible, of course, that instead of a mysterious "youth hormone" being contributed by the young rat to the old, the young rat's blood merely helps to dilute and draw off some of the "death hormones" circulating in the blood of the old rat. If some of the deleterious substances are being drawn off into the bloodstreams of the younger rats, should this not expose their cells to the ravages of the death hormones sooner than would otherwise have been the case? They should therefore have grown old faster than *their* littermates. Did they? Unfortunately, the results do not yet provide a clear-cut answer. This answer, and many more, should emerge from the research of Bar Harbor's David Harrison, who now has plans for an ambitious series of parabiotic mouse experiments.

The same questions about the presence of a possible hormonal youth factor were raised by scientists like Finch in interpreting experiments such as Krohn's serial skin transplants. Though these do not strictly represent parabiosis, which normally applies to the joining of whole animals rather than the transplantation of cells, those cells are nevertheless nourished by the bloodstream of their younger hosts, and their life spans consequently prolonged.

And now let us examine what all this has to do with genetic switches.

Chapter XIII

THE PROTEINS
THAT SWITCH GENES ON
AND OFF

From all the aging "experiments" described in the foregoing two chapters—nature's accelerations with the Pacific salmon and human progeria, and our decelerations via cooling, calorie restriction, and parabiosis—it is clear that (1) the rate of aging can be influenced by various circumstances, and (2) there is a complex interplay between organismic aging and cellular aging. As we know, a cell in culture ages and dies in a different manner, and at a different pace, than the same cell when it is a component of an organism.

Inasmuch as many-celled organisms are believed to have evolved from single-celled organisms, it is reasonable to expect each cell to retain, in some measure, the capacity for running through a life cycle possessed by the cell when it was a separate, independent being. It also makes sense that the cell's capabilities, in the context of the larger body of which it has become a part, would be subordinate to that organism's central controls; otherwise how could the organism develop into what it needs to become? The central controls, usually hormonal, would in most cases prevail. But in the absence, or failure to function, of those controls, the cell would proceed with the program it never lost, modified though it may have become in the course of its evolution. This is what seems to occur *in vitro,* when cells are freed from their usual constraints.

In the experiments in insect development which Joan Whitten carried out at Northwestern, she demonstrated that cell death, during the early part of the life cycle, could come about either in response to hormonal command, or as a result of "clocked" death mechanisms within the cell's nucleus. It does look more and more as if there might be at least two clocks of aging—the cell's own, carried somewhere in its nuclear molecular lattices, and the brain's hypothalamic-pituitary hormone chronometer. Moreover, it is clear that hormones can act on individual cells just as readily at the nuclear level as at the cytoplasmic. As one example cited by James H. Clark of the Baylor College of Medicine in Houston, based on his own research, steroid hormones—e.g., estrogen, hydrocortisone—are known to be capable of acting directly on the chromosomes to alter the nature and timing of gene transcription. In the absence of such interference, the cell follows its own internal clock. Thus Hayflick and Denckla could both be right, as already suggested. It also looks as if, regardless of *what* triggers the pattern of nuclear events, which in turn express themselves as degenerative changes, the events themselves come to pass by virtue of the turning on and off of genetic switches, the repression and de-repression of those pieces of information that govern all the cell's activities at any given moment in life. Our return to genetic on-off switches makes it appear—again—that Strehler, too, is right. (The names of Hayflick, Denckla, and Strehler are used here once more to symbolize the strongly held views which they represent. They do of course share these views with other investigators.)

The heart of the gerontological enterprise, then, may be to learn how these switches are turned on and off—and how to control them for our own benefit. This assumes, as discussed earlier, that the genetic information is not destroyed or damaged but rather masked, covered up, repressed, unavailable. For certain purposes we would like to de-repress it, to uncover it. At times it would of course be handy to know how to re-repress—as in the unregulated division of cancer cells. In fact, before we ever used the capacity to de-repress artificially, we would want to be sure we were able to re-repress when we had had enough of whatever activity we had turned on again—just as we would never build a nuclear reactor without feeling certain that we would turn it off whenever it threatened to "go critical."

In my discussions of genetic on-off switching—gene expression and gene regulation are other ways of saying the same thing—I have so far not emphasized sufficiently that the chromosomes are actually *nucleoproteins*. That is, they are made up not only of DNA but also of associated proteins (though those proteins are originally manufactured in the cytoplasm), and, at times, some RNA as well. I have also avoided spelling out the celebrated "operon theory" promulgated by the Nobel prize team of Jacques Monod and François Jacob of the Pasteur Institute in Paris; not because it is too devilishly complicated to explain—many people have successfully explained it, including Monod and Jacob themselves (in an elegant review article in the *Journal of Molecular Biology*)—but rather because it requires the acquisition of terminology which is not really necessary to the pursuit of our major themes. It should be known, however, that these were the two theorists and investigators who contributed the "breakthrough" concepts that enabled us to understand (insofar as we do understand it) the nature of genetic on-off switching. Research over the past few years has brought new understanding, especially of the role of the nucleoproteins in gene regulation. These more recent insights, and the evidence for them, are carefully spelled out in a 1975 *Scientific American* article by Gary S. Stein and Janet Swinehart Stein of the University of Florida, in collaboration with Lewis J. Kleinsmith of the University of Michigan.

In an earlier chapter, we did briefly consider that class of nucleoproteins known as *histones,* which James Bonner, Holger von Hahn, and others—notably Rockefeller University's Vincent G. Allfrey and Alfred E. Mirsky—have demonstrated to be the repressor proteins, the off switches. The histones literally cover the segments of DNA which contain the information that is meant to be Off Limits for the messenger-RNA molecules charged with the job of transcribing the information. In fact, when that information is suppressed, the manufacture of the messenger-RNA molecules also comes to a halt. We will recall that Robert T. Simpson of NIH had speculated that the tightness of the histone bonds, which kept that part of the DNA folded up like an accordion which therefore could not make music, is what repressed the information; while the loosening up of the histones is what permitted the accordion to play again. But what loosens up the histones? Simpson's theory implied that the histones did it themselves. But, as it turns out, they cannot do this without the assistance of the *nonhistone* nucleoproteins, which come in a profusion of varieties and possess enormous versatility.

Histones do not, as originally thought, possess the ability to recognize specific gene sites—as, say, an antibody recognizes an antigen, or a piece of transfer RNA recognizes an amino acid. They rather have a generalized ability to cover up any part of the DNA, just as a layer of putty can be slapped over any surface, regardless of its detailed configurations; or as a plastic barrier can deny access to a bookshelf without having to conform to the contours of the books or "know" anything about the books' contents or why they are not to be approached. The quantity of histones remains stable, too—just enough to cover up all the genetic information on all the DNA molecules. The nonhistones, on the other hand, vary considerably in their presence at any given moment—often depending on the number of genes that are turned on or off and the quantity of messenger-RNA molecules that are on hand. Some varieties of nonhistone protein seem unquestionably to serve important functions in gene regulation. They act as if they were equipped with an intelligent understanding of the scheduled details of the genetic program. At the appropriate time, and as if with purposive intent, they proceed to the segments of DNA which are ready to be de-repressed; by loosening the histone bonds (peeling back the layer of putty, taking the plastic barrier off the bookshelf), they render the genetic information accessible for use again, allowing the messenger RNA molecules to be made, and the RNA to transcribe and transmit the information.

In a series of experiments carried out by F. Marott Sinex and his associates at the Boston University School of Medicine, chromatin—which includes the DNA as well as the nucleoproteins—was separated from the nuclei of mouse-brain cells of varying ages. After meticulously eliminating all irrelevant substances, the leftover insoluble residues indicated the presence of increasing quantities of protein bound to the DNA as the mice aged. Nikitin, using a different set of techniques and a different set of cells (liver cells from albino rats), reported three consistent sets of results with age: (1) the number of repressors (histones) increases; (2) the number of derepressors (nonhistones) decreases; and (3) the making of chromatin RNA decreases. This strongly suggests that many more genes are turned *off* in the aging cell.

The very active role played by the nonhistones gives rise to an interesting speculation. In recent histories of the rise of molecular biology (all histories of this new enterprise must, of course, be recent), the historians like to point out how logical it was, in the beginning, to assume that the proteins were the chemicals of primary importance in the chromosomes. Proteins are so complex and versatile, having twenty different amino acids to draw upon, with virtually infinite combinations and arrangements; while the DNA, with its monotonous sequences and four-letter code, seemed to have many fewer possibilities.

Then came a whole series of discoveries: The truly epochal experiments of Rockefeller's Oswald T. Avery—who, somehow, never got the Nobel prize—which proved that it was DNA that contained the basic genetic information; the elucidation of the double helix by Crick and Watson; the insightful elaborations contributed by Monod and Jacob; the cracking of the genetic code by Marshall Nirenberg, Severo Ochoa, and others; and the rest of the book of molecular revelations. Now that everyone knows that DNA is the master molecule, we smile to think that we all once believed that protein was paramount.

Do we smile too soon? Consider: DNA does of course constitute the genetic manual of instructions—but does that make it the master? It is the library—but is it the librarian?

It would appear that the true intelligence in gene regulation lies in certain of the nonhistone proteins. If these are in fact the knowledgeable molecules charged with carrying out the genetic program, using a passive DNA as a convenient filing system or blueprint to be used only at the time and to the extent such use is appropriate, then it is the protein that is paramount after all. Of course, there do exist regulator genes, including repressor genes, that dictate the manufacture of the repressor proteins. But what turns the regulator genes on and off?

"It may not be long," say the Steins and Kleinsmith in *Scientific American,* "before proteins that regulate the expression of specific genes are isolated, introducing the possibility of a certain kind of genetic engineering: the proteins might be inserted into cells in order to modify abnormalities in gene transcription associated with development, differentiation and a broad spectrum of diseases, including cancer. Such a capability might revolutionize man's ability to deal with some profoundly destructive disorders."

It might also be one of the instruments which empower us to put an end to old age.

Chapter *XIV*

HOW AND WHEN IT MIGHT BEGIN TO HAPPEN

Just about the time I was arriving at this point in the book, and trying to look ahead a few chapters, I wrote to a doctor who I knew concerned himself officially with the social consequences of longevity on behalf of one of the state departments of health. I asked him if he might help me speculate about the consequences of an increased life span. His reply was thoughtful and useful within the scope of longevity problems as currently defined—those created mainly by the ever-increasing proportions of the population who are reaching old age. But he readily admitted, "I have not dealt with the hypothesis you raise, that in fact longevity will be increased," which he regarded an "unlikely event." He was even more explicit: "While speculation on the effects that increasing life span would have is fascinating, you will realize that most physicians believe it is in the realm of science fiction, rather than a practical possibility." He was neither chiding nor chastising me, simply pointing out, in a gentle, kindly way, a fact I might not be aware of.

But we have reached a point in our understanding when such complete skepticism—justified in the past—is rapidly becoming untenable. I do hope that, by now, I have offered sufficiently persuasive evidence and arguments to convince you that the possibility of an extended human life span has moved outside the realm of science fiction. It did belong in that realm until recently—just as going to the moon did, until recently. But no longer.

Let us examine, then, how soon we might hope to acquire the necessary knowledge; in what order we might expect the useful discoveries to arrive; and what the steps are in which we are likely to see the knowledge begin to be applied for our practical benefit, in terms of added good years of life.

It would be fatuous to forecast a precise timetable of developments. Too much depends on the availability of research funds, the creative limitations of individual investigators, good or bad luck, unforeseen obstacles. But we may feasibly hope that, with a bit of good luck and not too much bad luck, modest breakthroughs will begin to occur within a few decades. Strehler has guessed that we might know the essential answers before this century is out; but Hayflick believes that, in view of the resources being devoted to gerontology compared to the immeasurably larger sums going to other areas of research, Strehler's guess is too optimistic. Both men agree, though, that we fortunately do not have to wait until we know everything about the aging process in order to take advantage of what we do know. Jenner developed his smallpox vaccination without ever understanding much about why or how immunization occurred. We do not yet altogether understand the precise mechanisms of many common medications and therapies—aspirin is one example —which have been in everyday use for a long time.

Because research will proceed on many fronts and on many levels simultaneously, it is doubtful that practical applications will come in any orderly, step-by-step sequence. For an indefinite period, while gerontologists seek the more comprehensive answers, we will continue to do what medicine has sought to do all along: to cure or prevent specific diseases or palliate their symptoms; to combat or hold off the ravages of wear and tear in whatever piecemeal fashion presents itself.

Perhaps the most significant advances we could realistically hope for in the immediate future, in terms of an increased life expectancy, would be the conquest of the major killer diseases—the cardiovascular ailments and cancer. This is not to say that crash programs dedicated to those specific ends would be the most sensible or most economical way to attack the remaining degenerative diseases. The basic answers might sooner be attained through gerontological research than through research specifically labeled and designed to combat individual diseases.

Even after the basic gerontological questions have been answered, wear and tear may still remain our most persistent aging problem. If we had at hand, right now, the control mechanisms for all the genetic clocks, and could effectively employ these controls, our bodies and the individual cells within them would still be subject to the wear and tear that goes with mere existence in the world. To be sure—as already pointed out—if we had the secret of the genetic on-off switches at our command, we could hope to keep our self-repair functions operating for essentially indefinite time spans. Even so, we might have to find external methods of coping with some types of damage and erosion. The fortunate paradox is that wear and tear, which might be one of the last aging problems we overcome, is also one of the first we can begin to take effective measures against.

Biomedical scientists of all persuasions will of course continue to seek new surgeries, new medicines, new treatments, new vaccines, new theoretical approaches. To replace worn-out parts, transplantation techniques will be perfected and the immunological barrier overcome; and ever more sophisticated artificial replacements will be created. A concomitant hope is that the human body can be taught to regenerate its own missing or malfunctioning parts, as some other creatures do. But this kind of achievement is also likely to require a meticulous control of the appropriate genetic on-off switches. As for specific anti-aging therapies, several drugs already exist and are undergoing animal testing—in some cases, even limited human testing.

We earlier noted, for example, the gradual accumulation, over the years, of unsatisfactorily disposed of cellular garbage, especially the dark, fatty "old age pigment" called lipofuscin. It is found most plentifully, as might be expected, in nerve and muscle cells, which do not renew themselves after maturity. They do not have the advantage of cells which go on dividing; in mitotic cells, waste matter is continually diffused throughout the constantly self-renewing cellular bodies.

Few investigators look upon lipofuscin as a cause of aging, though most believe it is certainly a symptom of aging—probably harmless through most of life. As the wastes take up more and more of the cellular spaces, however, particularly in neurons, they may well interfere with cell functions, and therefore with overall mental activity. Can the wastes be cleared away, or prevented from forming in the first place?

There is no common agreement yet as to what causes lipofuscin to form, though many are convinced it must be the result of oxidation reactions, which turn loose free radicals to do their various kinds of damage, including the cross-linking of molecules inside the cell as well as outside it—e.g., in the connective tissue's collagen molecules. In that case, anything that might combat or correct free radical damage, or mop up free radicals before they can wreak their mischief, might be expected to reduce lipofuscin accumulations as well. Much of the lipofuscin seems to accumulate in the membranes of the cell's mitochondria, but a good bit of it may end up in the organelles known as *lysosomes*—little mentioned heretofore—which, among other functions, serve as the cells' garbage-disposal units. At least such is the view of Strehler, as well as Rockefeller University's Christian de Duve, who recently won a Nobel for his discovery of the lysosome.

When lysosomal membranes are damaged, harmful substances leaking through them may be responsible for many aging changes. This is the view of Richard Hochschild, who carries out his aging research under the unorthodox aegis of the Microwave Instrument Company in Corona del Mar, California. Acting on this hunch, Hochschild decided to try a natural substance called DMAE (for dimethylaminoethanol) as a possible retarder of senescence, because DMAE is known to be a lysosome membrane stabilizer. By adding DMAE to the drinking water of mice, Hochschild was able to increase their life spans significantly. Other investigators, notably Kalidas Nandy of Emory University in Atlanta (who has just moved to the Veterans Administration Hospital in Bedford, Massachusetts), have successfully employed a synthetic compound derived in part from DMAE—centrophenoxine (also known as meclofenoxate)— to retard the formation of lipofuscin in the brains of guinea pigs. In France, where centrophenoxine was first synthesized and shown to have almost no toxic side effects, the drug has been used experimentally, with apparent success, to improve the impaired mental capacities of senile human patients.

Other such drugs have been tried, with varying degrees of success reported. One such is vincamine (recently synthesized at the University of Rochester), a compound derived from the periwinkle plant; it seems to bolster the faltering intellectual abilities of patients with cerebrovascular disorders. Much more dramatic claims have been made for the well-publicized drug Gerovital (H3), developed by Ana Aslan of the Bucharest Geriatric Institute; but Gerovital has failed to gain acceptance in the United States.

"The apparent reversal of lipofuscin deposition [by centrophenoxine] is fascinating, and," in the opinion of Northwestern's Paul

Gordon, "indicates that latent lipofuscin scavenging mechanisms may be activated, to the advantage of the aging organism." Just as he believes centrophenoxine may trigger the cell's own latent capacities rather than attack lipofuscin as a direct garbage-cleanup agent, so does Gordon believe that Hochschild's DMAE may simply activate or enhance the cell's self-repair mechanisms rather than plugging the leaks in the lysosomal membranes. Gordon has himself been experimenting with yet another drug related to DMAE— isoprinosine (or methisoprinol)—and finds that it "partially reverses the deteriorated brain functioning of aged rats."

Previous chapters have already emphasized the effectiveness of various antioxidant substances in counteracting free radical damage. Jaime Miquel of NASA's Ames Laboratory in California has increased the life span of flies with antioxidants, while Harman and Tappel have done the same in mice. Meanwhile Kohn in Cleveland and Bjorksten in Madison have been testing, with some preliminary success, substances which appear to undo collagen damage and to inhibit cross-linkage.

There is already available, then, a varied array of potentially useful drugs, and this account does not begin to represent a complete sampling of the catalog of lipofuscin and cross-link inhibitors, antioxidants, immuno-regulators, hormones (including, of course, thymosin), coolants, and other agents which offer real hope of alleviating or retarding, at least temporarily and partially, many of the deleterious effects of aging. A number of pharmaceutical houses are of course following these experiments; some are actively engaged in them. A few excellent reviews of gerontologically promising drugs have been written by Charles G. Kormendy and A. Douglas Bender of the Smith, Kline & French Laboratories in Philadelphia. (Kormendy is now with Bristol Laboratories in Syracuse, New York.)

Some of the experimental substances are clearly testable in the almost immediate future. It could certainly be established with reasonable speed, as Comfort, Harman, and Hayflick have pointed out, whether or not antioxidants might be truly effective as anti-aging therapy and which antioxidants are the safest and most potent. Such research would not have to wait for any new basic information to come in.

Many experimental drugs, such as the unnamed temperature-lowering compound used by Rosenberg and Kemeny, have had such erratic side effects that they will undoubtedly require a long period of testing in animals before anyone is willing to try them on people.

Centrophenoxine, on the other hand, because of its relative freedom from adverse side effects, is likely to be tried soon on human patients in this country, as it has already in Europe. But its potential is not as great. Inasmuch as lipofuscin is not believed to cause any real harm until those senile years when mental faculties begin to fall off badly, its inhibition would supply only limited benefits. And if antioxidant therapy were to prove effective as an inhibitor of free radical damage, then it would probably serve as an inhibitor of lipofuscin formation as well.

Thymosin, which is already undergoing human testing in cancer and the immuno-deficiency diseases, is another likely candidate for anti-aging trials. Its importance will depend on how vital it is to the aging organism to maintain a high level of cell-mediated immunity.

In studying the proportions of various neurotransmitters present in the brain at any given time, Paola Timiras and Paul Segall at UC/Berkeley discovered—as already reported—rising levels of serotonin with age; but they also discovered that levels of dopamine go *down*. And indeed George Cotzias and his associates at Brookhaven have used L-dopa (developed as a medication for Parkinsonism), which stimulates dopamine production, to retard aging in laboratory animals. So now L-dopa may be added to the list of potential anti-aging drugs.

Some purely dietary therapies now outside the boundaries of conventional scientific interest—such as the regimen suggested by Benjamin Frank, whose work will be discussed briefly in the next chapter—may, as time goes on, earn more attention from the geriatric and gerontological community. Frank claims anti-aging benefits—and believes he has sound theoretical bases for his observed results—from a diet rich in nucleic acids, enzyme-activating vitamins, and proteins, sometimes supplemented by antioxidants. He emphasizes the importance of taking in these substances in a single meal so that everything needed for protein synthesis in the cells is supplied simultaneously.

At Chebotarev's institute in Kiev, gerontologists have been much readier than most American scientists to test the possible efficacy of unorthodox remedies, among them that highly nutritious secretion of the honeybee's pharyngeal glands known as "royal jelly" (because it is fed to all queen larvae); Ana Aslan's 2 per cent novocaine injections, best known outside Rumania as H3 or Gerovital; and

Academician V. P. Filatov's "tissue therapy"—which, with its use of placental tissue, somewhat resembles Swiss cellular therapy. The Kiev group has also concocted a number of experimental mixtures of their own, including a multivitamin complex they have named Decamevit (already in wide use in the U.S.S.R.) and a hormonal preparation called Nerobol. In addition, I. I. Brekham, a physiologist at the Institute of Marine Biology in Vladivostok, has found merit in the extracts of the wild plant *Eleutherococcus senticosus,* which, because of its family relationship to ginseng—whose root produces the time-honored Chinese and Korean tonic of that name— is known in the United States as Siberian ginseng. The only American investigator, to my knowledge, who is looking into the anti-aging potential of *Eleutherococcus* is Boston's Marott Sinex.

Though the Russian researchers have reported good results in terms of improving the health and mental capacities of the aged with a number of these preparations, they are cautious about the indiscriminate use of such tonics and stimulants until they are better understood. In Chebotarev's own words: "It should be stressed . . . that there is as yet no sufficiently explicit, objective information pertaining to the pharmacodynamics of these agents, to their indication for the use in the treatment of the aged." Nevertheless, in view of the number of drugs now being prescribed—from digitalis to reserpine—which were originally herbal folk remedies, science should not disdain to investigate thoroughly substances that do seem to do some good.

Hayflick has suggested that some daring, spartan types might want to try out McCay's calorie-restriction experiments on themselves in the interests of a longer life span. He doubts it, though, on the grounds that in the forty years since McCay published his original results, no one has yet tried it; and from this apparent lack of interest has drawn the conclusion that "for most people the quality of life is more important than its quantity," and that, if this is so, "any method that might increase human longevity is unacceptable even if it minimally affects the enjoyment of life."

I believe this is a premature conclusion. Though McCay's work has been in the literature for forty years, the general public has not heard much about it. Moreover, whoever were to make such a decision would have to make it before puberty—not usually considered the age of informed consent—and would have to stay with it essentially forever, no minor feat of self-discipline. And who would venture to predict with any assurance that the data from rats would be translatable to human beings, or that it would be safe? Anyone taking the long gamble would have to know that all the deprivation might be wasted, might in fact be harmful. Even so, I am convinced that if one could start such a regimen later in life, with reasonable assurance of safety and a longer life, many would volunteer. Timiras and Segall believe that—unlike the McCay calorie-restricted diet that must be started before puberty—their tryptophan-restricted diet may work at later stages of life as well, in which case we might get a chance to test people's motivation. For the moment of course, this must all remain in the realm of pure speculative psychology.

A vast amount of literature has been accumulated on the biochemical consequences of aging. Kanungo, for example, in a long review article in *Biochemical Reviews,* lists dozens of such aging changes. Enzyme levels may be especially important as indicators of the aging process. The quantity and activity of hundreds of different kinds of enzymes change with age. If it becomes known with certainty that the absence or lowered activity of identifiable enzymes is responsible for loss of function, then perhaps those enzymes or enzyme activators can be supplied artificially either orally or by injection. If, on the other hand, functional loss is invariably associated with an increase in either the quantity or activity of various other enzymes, then perhaps specific inhibitors can be found for those enzymes. Thus one can envision a kind of enzyme and anti-enzyme cocktail mix or injection as an anti-aging treatment—though each ingredient would have to be added with great care, with sure knowledge of its role in aging. An indiscriminate mixture of enzymes might supply some that were already in oversupply and thus accelerate aging.

Enzyme replacement therapy has already been tried on a limited basis for certain genetic diseases. Roscoe Brady and his associates at the National Institute of Neurological Diseases and Stroke have been pioneers in this field. There are two genetic disorders—Fabry's disease and Gaucher's disease—both of which can cause widespread damage and suffering, and usually premature death, in their victims. Each is caused by a single missing enzyme responsible for one step of breaking down a particular molecule. Failure at that step brings the breakdown process to a halt; hence harmful substances accumulate in vital tissues and organs.

Brady and his team painstakingly extracted and purified both enzymes over a period of years from human placentas. Unfortunately, the supply was too small to carry out the treatments for very long, but they were able to prove that injection of the missing enzymes into victims of these diseases did in fact alleviate symptoms and measurably reduce the accumulations of the substance that was their target. Many feel that these experiments of Brady's, reported at length in the *New England Journal of Medicine,* hold out great hope for the hundred-or-so genetic diseases that have been identified as enzyme disorders. There is no reason why, if it works, similar enzyme therapy could not be applied to declining cell function with aging.

One possibility that worried Brady in carrying out these experiments was that his enzyme injections—since they were in a sense implantations of foreign protein—might activate the body's immune system into rejecting the replacement enzymes and nullifying the treatment, especially if the therapy were to be carried out on a long-term basis. This same concern was strongly expressed in an article by three Johns Hopkins scientists—Samuel H. Boyer, David C. Siggers, and Leslie J. Krueger—in *The Lancet.* They warned that a potent immune reaction could even cause death; but they did propose tests by which patients who were especially at risk in this regard might be detected.

Meanwhile a new and more reliable technique of enzyme delivery has been devised that might circumvent this problem altogether. Among those pursuing this truly exciting possibility are Gerald Weissmann of New York University, its principal inventor; Ernest Beutler of the City of Hope Medical Center at Duarte, California; Beutler's former colleague, Satish Srivastava, now carrying out a vigorous independent program at UTMB/Galveston; Gregory Gregoriadis of the Clinical Research Center at Harrow, England; and, again, Abe White of Stanford and Syntex. These investigators have been working with *liposomes* (a term coined by Weissmann), tiny biodegradable spheres of fatty material in which enzymes can be trapped and transported through the circulatory system and protected from reacting with the body's own substances until they arrive at some point close to the target sites.

How ensure that the liposomes, the messengers carrying their precious freight of enzymes, get into the cells that need them? It occurred to NYU's Weissmann and his associates that one type of

cell, the *leukocyte,* has access to every part of the body. The leukocyte is the white blood cell that carries out phagocytic activities,
engulfing any "enemy" material it encounters. Could leukocytes
somehow be induced to engulf the enzyme-carrying liposomes and
transport them to the desired cells—particularly to brain and nerve
cells, where the enzyme deficiency does its damage in such genetic
afflictions as Tay-Sachs disease? It turned out that they could.
When a liposome is coated with a special immunoglobulin devised
by Weissmann, it becomes a would-be friend which must however
masquerade as an enemy in order to carry out its benign mission.
The leukocyte, fooled by the disguise, engulfs the liposome and carries it along to the defective cell.

What was needed to test the concept was an experimental animal
whose cells were totally deficient in a given enzyme which could be
supplied from the outside. If you can find the enzyme in a given
quantity in a cell which normally has none at all, then all ambiguity
as to how it got there has been removed. Weissmann, working at the
marine biological laboratories at Woods Hole, found the smooth
dogfish *Mustelus canis* ideal for his purposes; its cells altogether lack
the class of enzymes known as peroxidases. Encapsulating horse-
radish peroxidase in liposomes, and using the method described,
Weissmann found that the dogfish's cells took up as much as 50
per cent of the enzymes within a period of 60 hours—impressive
indeed when compared with Brady's earlier technique, where the
target cells finally received no more than one tenth of one per cent
of the injected enzymes.

By now—at NYU, at City of Hope, and at Galveston—human
Tay-Sachs cells have been "cured" *in vitro* by using these new
techniques. There are some thirty or more such genetic "lysosomal
storage diseases" (the unwanted product accumulates in the lysosomes because the enzyme required to break it down is absent) in
which a single missing enzyme has been implicated. Weissmann and
Srivastava both agree that liposome encapsulation as a means of
enzyme replacement promises a feasible treatment method in all
these diseases.

There is no reason, of course, why liposome encapsulation need
be confined to enzyme therapy. Gregoriadis, at Harrow, has experi-
mented with entrapping other kinds of protein in liposomes and
thus avoiding allergic reactions. He has explored the drug-carrying
potentials of liposomes in cancer chemotherapy, and done research

which suggests that enzymes entrapped in liposomes could pass through the bloodstream without attracting the attention of antibodies and would only be liberated in the liver and spleen. He further suggests that liposomes might carry fragments of DNA and RNA when necessary.

As an alternative to using enzymes, natural or synthetic, as replacement therapy, Bibudhendra Sarkar at The Hospital for Sick Children in Toronto has suggested that one could pinpoint the active sites of certain enzymes—choosing the site which represents the essential function in which one is interested—and manufacture tiny molecules that *mimic* that particular function. "It may be possible," he says, in Upjohn's *Guidelines to Metabolic Therapy,* "to design the active site of an enzyme that is missing in an individual suffering from a genetic disorder and administer the synthetic molecule as a substitute." Sarkar has succeeded in synthesizing such a compound; it mimics the copper transport site on human albumin. In this instance, his synthetic molecule was only one four-thousandth as complex as the albumin molecule itself! How might it be used? In Wilson's disease, an inherited and sometimes fatal defect of copper metabolism, this miniature mimic might be employed to remove the excess copper which otherwise accumulates in the brain, kidney, liver, and red blood cells of the victim. At times, "when a larger molecule is needed for specific purposes," says Sarkar, "the synthesized active site may be attached to any convenient molecule," and, sent into the body as a piggyback rider, could do the job that would ordinarily require the whole molecule. Here again there is no theoretical reason why such replacement techniques could not be used in anti-aging therapy.

Many methods could of course be used in combinations that would deal symptomatically with the observable and measurable consequences of the aging process—such as some of the compounds being investigated by the Russians. Such therapy would be particularly important if the treated consequences in turn had other consequences, which often seems to be the case. This cascade effect, as Finch would call it, has been worked out mathematically by Strehler and A. S. Mildvan in a well-known but complex theory that predicts the decline in an organism's "viability index," based on the total impact of all the aging factors that influence it. Many purely symptomatic treatments could well have the effect of keeping our viability index much higher for much longer periods of time.

In the end, though, no matter how many antidotes we find for specific kinds of wear and tear, no matter how many diseases we cure or prevent, if we do nothing about the basic aging process, we will still die when our genetic program runs out. Hayflick envisions people who had not even been ill suddenly dropping dead at the age of, say, one hundred—going all at once, like "the wonderful one-hoss shay." He considers this a laudable outcome, however, as does René Dubos. Dubos has some doubts about the wisdom, or even the morality, of extending the human life span, but feels it would be an unmitigated good to keep people in the best of health through all the years for which they were programmed. To keep people fully functional and in possession of all their faculties until the very end is the noncontroversial goal of gerontology, conforming with the stated aim of the Gerontological Society to add life to years rather than years to life.

Nevertheless, many gerontologists, and many of the citizens who support their work, will not want to stop there. And it may be unreasonable as well as undesirable, as knowledge accumulates, to expect them to stop there. A major goal—despite its controversial aspects—is still the real extension of the human life span for significant periods of time.

If Denckla is right about a hormonal clock of aging, then his quest, if it is crowned with success, certainly moves us in that direction. His plan is, first, to isolate and synthesize the death hormone, then to create an anti-death hormone that would destroy it and counteract its influence—a tedious business at best, even if findings fit theories. There may be a shortcut, however. Once the death hormone is better identified, we will be better able to identify the releasing factor by which the hypothalamus instructs the pituitary to produce the hormone. There appears to be a separate releasing factor (RF) for every pituitary hormone. The RFs thus far discovered, principally by Guillemin, are much smaller and simpler molecules than the pituitary hormones they control. Thus, instead of having to synthesize a complex hormone and create an equally complex inhibitor, we could hope to work with the RF and find a substance that inhibits *its* release by the hypothalamus. This would enormously simplify the task—though it could still not be called a simple task. In any case, the end result would be that death hormones would not be released by the pituitary, and the programmed blockade of thyroid hormone would not come to pass; hence cells would not age, except for the overlay of wear-and-tear damage—which, by then, might or might not have been largely overcome.

If we were able in this manner to abort the hormonal clock, that would be one genetic program down—but perhaps one still to go: the cell's own nuclear genetic clock. To affect this in any substantial way would require genetic manipulation, or "genetic engineering," which many see as too far off in the future (if ever, indeed, it becomes possible at all) to incorporate into any of our plans or expectations.

This judgment, too, is premature—and is of course not universally shared. A stance of overriding pessimism is simply not warranted in the face of the startling cellular events that have taken place in so many laboratories around the world.

Chapter XV

GENE TRANSPLANTS AND SHORTCUTS TO TESTING

The experiments of William F. Munyon at Buffalo's Roswell Park Memorial Institute may serve as one random example of genetic engineering already at work in laboratory situations. In an earlier chapter, I made passing mention of embryonic substances that reappear in the adult afflicted with cancer. One of these substances is the enzyme thymidine kinase (TK). The fact that TK seems to resurface only in cancer victims suggests that it might have something to do with stimulating nondividing cells to begin dividing again. Munyon was able to transfer the gene for TK from the herpes simplex virus to nondividing mouse cells *in vitro*—and the mouse cells were thenceforth able to divide again! Munyon's results were confirmed by Richard Davidson of the Harvard Medical School, who further discovered that TK production was shut down after some sixty to eighty generations (the Hayflick limit?). Davidson was also able to ascertain that the TK gene was not lost at that point, but merely repressed—and therefore could conceivably be de-repressed. What has already been achieved suggests that we may not be too far from that kind of knowledge.

Frank Ruddle of Yale, by fusing a mouse liver-tumor cell to a human lymphocyte, transferred genetic material which enabled the lymphocyte to make albumin. The transferred substance, in this case, may have merely activated a gene already present but never used, since lymphocytes have no need to synthesize albumin. Whether the occurrence represents the turning on of a genetic switch, or an actual gene transplant, it certainly qualifies as a piece of genetic engineering. "We're still a long, long way from being able to carry out such repair functions in humans, or even in experimental animals for that matter," says Ruddle—who has performed numerous genetic engineering feats via cell fusion and hybridization—in *Medical World News*. "But unquestionably the possibilities are there, and, as we develop a more sophisticated knowledge of human and mammalian genetics through these somatic cell systems, we will perceive opportunities for successfully carrying out gene grafting." Paul Berg of Stanford is one of many biologists working in these areas who believe it is quite feasible to hitch specific genes onto viruses, much as Sarkar hopes to hitch a tiny partial molecule onto a larger one, as a means of transporting the genes to the target cells.

Two experiments in genetic engineering are of special interest in terms of human disease:

In the genetic disorder galactosemia, an enzyme that enables the normal body to metabolize galactose is missing. If the deficiency is detected in infancy, the victim's lot can be greatly improved by putting him on a milk-free diet. But galactosemia can be a serious disease, indeed a fatal one. In 1971, Carl R. Merril of the National Institute of Mental Health—working with a pair of NIH colleagues, Mark R. Geier and John C. Petricciani—found that a bacterial virus, the so-called lambda phage, was able to steal from *Escherichia coli* bacteria the gene that coded for the missing enzyme. In a series of experiments which *Nature* hailed as "little short of revolutionary," Merril and his associates took skin cells from a human galactosemia victim and exposed them to lambda phage in tissue culture. The human cells, previously deficient in this respect, were then able to metabolize galactose. Moreover, succeeding generations of the cells kept the ability long after any viruses were around to provide the material.

This could only mean that the genetic information stolen from the bacteria had now been transferred to the human cells—and incorporated, as a permanent hereditary acquisition (thus an artificial mutation), into the genes of the formerly galactosemic cells. In tissue culture, at least, genetic engineering had cured a human disease, just as the enzyme replacement techniques of Weissmann and Srivastava had cured Tay-Sachs *in vitro*. Transferring the technique to whole persons will be a much more complex matter, but the possibility of genetic therapy has been clearly demonstrated. We can hope that other viruses might serve similarly as purveyors of stolen genetic goods—and, in such cases, none of us would mind being accessories after the fact, or even risk serving as "fences."

Nature, at the time it published the Merril report, warned: "It is inevitable that virtually all readers, having seen the title of this report ["Bacterial Virus Gene Expression in Human Cells"], will probably find their minds flooding with *a priori* scepticism and prejudice as they begin to read the text. And as Merril and his colleagues no doubt realize and must accept, everybody will be out to find flaws in their work." But, after a discussion of the experiments, the *Nature* editorial concluded that "even the most dyed-in-the-wool sceptics will be very hard put to it to find anything seriously wrong with the design and execution of these experiments."

Merril's results were indeed challenged on many sides. But soon his experiments, and similar ones with other types of cells, were being duplicated in a number of other laboratories. Ken Roozen and Douglas Jasper, after visiting Merril's lab at NIMH to observe his techniques, were able to carry out gene transplants of their own at the University of St. Louis. Roozen has now moved on to the University of Alabama Medical Center, where he is continuing his investigations. From Germany came Jurgen Horst who, on his return to the University of Freiburg, set up a series of experiments patterned after Merril's. With his Freiburg colleagues and Konrad Beyreuther of the University of Cologne, Horst again used the bacterial virus—the lambda phage—as the "transplant surgeon" and *E. coli* as the "donor" of the gene. But this time it was a different gene—the one carrying instructions for making the enzyme beta-galactosidase—because the "recipient" was different: cells taken from the victim of another genetic disease, a form of gangliosidosis which causes severe mental retardation due to a deficiency of that enzyme. The genetic surgery was a success. The transplant took. The viruses were able to "infect" the cells with the gene for making the enzyme, and the cells were thereafter able to make their own.

To Merril's lab also came Barry Rolfe from The National University of Australia in Canberra. Rolfe, too, was able to carry out the gene transplant that cured the galactosemic cells. Moreover, Rolfe and his colleagues have discovered that a species of gray kangaroo, *Macropus fuliginosus,* naturally has an enormously reduced level of the enzyme—since the animal doesn't need it—which is missing in human galactosemia victims. Hence a ready-made animal exists as an experimental model. Rolfe has already been able to induce higher production of the enzyme in *Macropus* by apparently transplanting genes—again the *E. coli* gene delivered by the same lambda phage. These experiments are barely beginning. Meanwhile other scientists in other nations are moving ahead on similar *in vitro* gene transplants, among them teams of investigators at the University of Brussels and the Bar Ilan University in Israel.

Nor has Merril's group stopped with that first experiment. One of Merril's collaborators, young Mark Geier—who only recently earned his doctorate—is eager to push ahead in the direction of curing or preventing human genetic diseases. Working with some graduate students at NIMH, he has devised two very promising model systems, in both cases starting out with normal mice. In the one instance, he feeds the mice lethal amounts of galactose, more than their bodies can handle, so that 80 per cent of them die within two weeks. But he can keep them living significantly longer by transferring the bacterial genes via the lambda phage so that their bodies are then capable of processing much of the *excess* galactose. So, in a sense, he has artificially produced galactosemia—and then partially cured it— in these mice.

A second set of mice were ingeniously *declared* to be abnormal in an important respect: they suffered from leucine deficiency. But so do all mammals. Leucine is simply one of the amino acids we take in with our protein foods. We cannot survive without it. Since our bodies cannot manufacture leucine, we may be said to suffer from a genetic leucine deficiency disease; or, as Merril puts it, "all of us have a lethal genetic defect which we treat daily by eating leucine." What Mark Geier has been doing is withholding from the mice their daily "medication." As a result, they die within a two-month period. Such is the sophistication, by now, in regard to the *E. coli*–lambda phage genetic-transplant system, that two other scientists at NIH were able to construct a lambda carrying the genes necessary for manufacturing leucine. Mice injected with this virus—even though they still get no leucine in their diets—live *seven months longer* than the control groups. In an animal with a life span of between one and two years, a seven-month extension can hardly be deemed insignificant. Thus have one set of imaginative experiments in Carl Merril's lab at NIMH resulted in a "cascade effect" of other genetic engineering feats around the world—feats which have already gone far beyond what anyone would have thought possible only a short time ago. (In fact, scientists who have not yet heard about these results still rate them as impossible.)

Let us look at one more experiment, since it is the first medical attempt at gene therapy, that is, the treatment of human patients by means of genetic-engineering techniques. In this case the carrier virus was the Shope papilloma virus, and the genetic disease was argininemia. This disorder had never been heard of before 1969. The name for it was coined by a German doctor, Heinz G. Terheggen of the University Pediatric Clinic in Cologne, to cover the basic defect in a mysterious ailment that afflicted two young sisters. Their blood arginine levels were ten times higher than normal, probably due to a hereditary lack of the enzyme arginase. Reading the report of these cases in *The Lancet,* Nobel geneticist Joshua Lederberg of Stanford called it to the attention of Stanfield Rogers at Oak Ridge (now at the University of Tennessee). He did so because he knew that Rogers had long been interested in the Shope papilloma virus, which produces nonmalignant skin growths in rabbits. One characteristic of the Shope virus is its ability to produce a form of arginase. In fact, laboratory technicians who had worked with the Shope virus were shown to have lower than normal blood arginine levels—an indicator that the virus's genetic material was functioning in human bodies, though apparently producing no ill effects.

So it looked as if Lederberg had perhaps discovered a disease to go with Stanfield Rogers's remedy. Rogers got in touch with Terheggen, who sent skin samples of the argininemic girls. Grown in tissue culture, the cells responded to challenge by the virus, and were able to produce arginase. The girls' doctors then decided to try the Shope virus as the only treatment that might possibly save the victims from otherwise certain death. The virus looked relatively safe—after forty years of experience with it and no known instance of human beings (even those known to be infected with it) suffering adverse effects. Even so, they used cautiously small doses of the virus (and were criticized for so doing). The treatment might be said to have worked, in that it did reduce the girls' blood arginine levels by some 20 per cent. But they were far gone by then, and died. It was apparently a case of too little and too late to help the unfortunate sisters. Nevertheless, exciting prospects have been opened up for genetic therapy in the future.

As an expression of faith in the commercial potential of genetic engineering, Britain's Imperial Chemical Industries, Ltd. (ICI), decided in 1974 to invest £ 40,000 in a three-year joint project with the University of Edinburgh, based on the research of Kenneth and Noreen Murray in the viral transmission of genes.

I could go on and on citing experimental examples which bolster my own conviction that if there is a genetic clock of aging, and if it is located in the cell's nucleus, we will sooner or later be able to manipulate it; and by "later," I don't mean the remotely distant future—though I could not begin to pin a date on the achievement.

Let us now move ahead a step and suppose that we already had at hand anti-aging chemicals, enzyme cocktails, "pacemaker" hormones (or counteractive anti-hormones) to regulate the rate of aging, or genetic engineering techniques, or any combination of these—thoroughly tested in the laboratory and found to possess no serious side effects. Such a supposition requires that we swallow some large assumptions. But, blithely ignoring all interim obstacles for the moment, let's do suppose the existence of this state of affairs. Even so, how could we test these therapies on people and, within a reasonable period of time, prove that the subjects' lives were truly being prolonged?

It would seem that we would have to wait an entire lifetime to see if a given individual died on schedule or not. And the criteria by which we could fix an arbitrary figure for anyone's "scheduled" life span would be difficult to establish. True, if enough people in a population began to live far longer—beyond any reasonable expectation—than members of the same population who were not getting anti-aging therapy, then we could begin to feel some confidence that the therapy was working. But it would surely require statistically significant quantities of people over several generations to prove both efficacy and safety, would it not? Under such circumstances, the gerontologists who started the project would not live to see the end of it—though they might gain some hope by secretly dosing themselves with the still untried elixir. And would the next generation of gerontologists care? Would the money continue to come forth to meet the expenses of such a large-scale undertaking over so long a time, especially if it was dependent on the vagaries of congressional appropriations? Exactly such considerations have often in the past discouraged biologists from entering this field of research. Investigators like to see the end results of their work; hence their preference for short-lived, quick-turnover species—*E. coli,* rotifers, *Drosophila,* or, at most, mice.

These temporal obstacles would pose formidable difficulties even for the dauntless. Fortunately, some realistic shortcuts may exist. Their success would depend on our ability to establish reliable measurements to determine an individual's rate of aging over relatively short periods of time. If we knew this, we might then test for a given therapy's effectiveness by monitoring the significant aging factors to see if their rate was indeed slowing down.

Such a battery of tests to determine aging changes in the short run has been proposed by Alex Comfort. In devising an array of tests, it would be important to select functions that could be counted on to decline steadily and irreversibly with age, though it should be emphasized that a decline in function might show up as an *increase* in a given substance. Measurements of parameters such as serum cholesterol levels and blood pressure would not do, therefore, because although these are factors usually associated with aging and degenerative diseases, they do not decline steadily; they rather tend to go up and down somewhat erratically during any given time period. The chosen functions would also have to decline in clearly measurable degrees over relatively short periods—say, three to five years—so that meaningful experiments could be carried out within that kind of time span. Comfort suggests that the subjects, at the start, be around fifty years old, and that they be men in order to "avoid further statistical breakdown and complications associated with differences in age of menopause, which affects some variables." A great deal of data on the decline of physiological functioning with aging has been gathered over the years in a number of longitudinal studies—that is, studies carried out with the same subjects over long stretches of time—especially a continuing study of hundreds of the same men who have been coming regularly, for many years, to GRC/Baltimore.

Though Comfort's original suggestion for the test battery was spelled out in a detailed technical article in *The Lancet,* he has explained his idea more briefly and simply in *Playboy:* ". . . we can now move into human studies, because greater knowledge of age changes and the advent of automated clinical laboratories and computers make it possible to measure the rate of aging in the short run.

"The new strategy is to choose a battery of measurements— chemical, psychological and clinical—that change with age and follow them over a period of, say, five years, starting at a given age, such as 50. The measures are picked to be so varied that any factor that slows the rate of change in all of them would be likely to act by slowing down aging in general. This approach reduces the problem of how to retard aging in man to the size of an ordinary medical experiment, using some 500 volunteers over three to five years, like the assessment of low-cholesterol diets in heart disease.

"Battery tests for aging are one of the few beneficent spin-offs from the bomb. They were developed at the Brookhaven nuclear-research laboratories to measure the rate of aging in Hiroshima survivors. (Reassuringly the survivors didn't age faster.) Equipment like that which would be needed to carry out such tests on normal people already exists in many U.S. centers, such as the Kaiser-Permanente Medical Centers in San Francisco, Oakland and Walnut Creek, California. We could start human experiments next week, measuring such things as hair graying, skin elasticity, change in body chemicals, hearing and mental agility as indexes of the speed at which aging is progressing."

Benjamin Schloss of Los Angeles has designed an elaborate "interaction chamber" (the prototype remains to be built) which would provide plenty of room for an individual to lie down comfortably in its carefully controlled interior. The subject, with face mask and numerous sensors and other instrumentation hooked up to a computer, could have enormous quantities of data about his physiological condition recorded and processed instantaneously. The chamber and its associated systems, Schloss believes, would enable him to measure the decrease in the functional capacities and response times of the whole body, as well as its various organs, tissues, and individual cells. His short-range objective is twofold: (1) "the determination of the nature of the deterioration by identifying those changes that are responsible for each type of deterioration"; and (2) "the application of corrective measures by introducing substances that compensate for the observed changes."

I say "short-range objective" because his longer-range aim, like that of Strehler, Hayflick, Denckla, and so many others, is to locate the regulators of the clock of aging, and to turn those regulators to our own uses. As an added interim measure, Schloss believes that Comfort's basic idea can be carried out in a much more sophisticated fashion at the biochemical level. Hundreds, perhaps thousands, of substances change in their quality and quantity as the organism ages, in Schloss's view, and an instant interpretation of these changes could probably be read in a single blood sample. There do now exist automated blood analyzers that, requiring only a drop of blood, routinely carry out a dozen or so blood tests simultaneously and return the answers in a minute or two. Would it really be possible to get such instant readings on hundreds, even thousands, of different substances in the same manner? Schloss's answer is positive. Schloss, whose training is more in biomedical engineering than in gerontology per se, has in fact obtained a patent on exactly such a device—though, again, a prototype has not yet been constructed. He insists, moreover, that the device is amazingly simple in its operational principles. Another device that aims to achieve similar feats—that is, offer instant readouts on hundreds of substances from a single blood sample, this one based on ultraviolet spectroscopy—is being developed by the Belgian biophysicist Frank J. G. Van den Bosch at SUNY's Downstate Medical Center in Brooklyn.

If these devices work as hoped, Schloss is convinced that a single blood sample could tell a great deal about the functions of the liver, kidney, and other organs, in terms of the chemicals they deposit into the bloodstream. What this means for aging research is that, if you can list 100, or 500, of the biochemical changes that take place with aging, then you can measure them all at once in a single person.

If you do this on a large number of people of different ages over a period of time, you can begin to establish a "biochemical profile" of a person whose average age is, say, thirty. (You will also in that case have a diagnostic early warning system in the event of any organ malfunction.) You can also quickly establish the individual's *rate* of aging over short periods of time, as Comfort hoped. Then you can readily tell if your pacemaker chemicals, your enzyme-cocktail mix, your genetic on-off switching devices, are slowing down his rate of aging or not.

Schloss's ideas, it should be emphasized, do not yet have any currency in the gerontological community, nor can they hope to until his machines can be built and his methods adequately tested. But the pessimism over the feasibility of testing anti-aging therapies without having to wait a lifetime is clearly giving way to a more hopeful outlook. When the medications and pacemaker substances are ready for human trials, methods may well be at hand for ascertaining their value, or lack of it, within reasonable time spans. Moreover, Alex Comfort sees no reason why anti-aging substances, once they are discovered, synthesized, tested, and put on the market, should not be just as universally available as any other drug or medical treatment.

They may, in fact, be cheaper and more available than many of today's heroic but high-cost biomedical technologies.

If such pacemaker substances do become available to us, will they really be able to reach and affect cells everywhere in our bodies? It is reasonable to imagine so. At least, they might well exert beneficial effects on every tissue reached by the bloodstream. Might skin wrinkles, then, be unwrinkled, old muscles made supple, and gray hair retransformed to brown or red or blond? It is all possible. The tissues of the female reproductive tract certainly rejuvenate with hormonal treatment. But what of those parts of the eye, for example, which the blood circulation doesn't reach? And what about the teeth? How far can even the most sophisticated dentistry carry us? These are problems that may of course require separate solutions. And though they seem simpler than the overall aging problem, they could take longer to work out—just as one can imagine a cure or preventive for cancer while we continue to be afflicted with the common cold.

Chapter XVI

LAST BARRIER:
THE DYING BRAIN

What people worry about most when they worry about parts that may go on aging while the rest of the body remains young is the prospect of a dimming brain. Not everyone, of course. There are always the irrepressibles, like George Bernard Shaw, who was able to write (in the preface to *Back to Methuselah*) at eighty-nine: "Physically I am failing: my senses, my locomotive powers, my memory, are decaying at a rate which threatens to make a Struldbrug of me if I persist in living; yet my mind feels capable of growth; for my curiosity is keener than ever. My soul goes marching on; and if the Life Force would give me a body as durable as my mind . . . I might begin a political career as a junior civil servant and evolve into a capable Cabinet minister in another hundred years or so." But for every still-buoyant intellect that is pushing ninety, there are dozens much younger whose mental functions are noticeably impaired. And long before this becomes apparent through any overt behavior, brain cells have begun to die off at an alarming rate.

Based on studies such as those that Harold Brody (now at SUNY/Buffalo) made at the University of Minnesota in the early 1950's—and others as early as the 1920's—it has been estimated that the average man or woman, after the age of thirty-five, begins to lose something like 100,000 unreproducible neurons a day, every day of every ensuing year of life. That is hardly a negligible quantity, even considering that we start out with some 10 billion neurons when the brain attains full growth. Some have speculated that the loss of neurons may itself considerably accelerate—or even be a major cause of—the rest of the body's aging. Others believe that brain-cell death is not so much programmed, or even the result of intrinsic wear-and-tear processes, as it is the consequence of increasing circulatory inefficiency with age. The further consequence is that brain cells, which are more dependent than most other cells on a plentiful, continuous supply of blood-borne oxygen, die off in larger quantities than elsewhere.

Brain-cell death has been given a wholly novel interpretation, however, by zoologist Richard Dawkins of Oxford. "It is a widely deplored fact," he wrote in *Nature* in 1971, "that every day many thousands of our brain cells die and, unlike other types of cell, are never replaced. I suggest that this may not be a purely destructive process, as is normally supposed. . . ." Dawkins proposed that neuron death may be a *selective* process, merely the visible manifestation of a purposive development of a most important brain function—the very "mechanism of information storage in the brain."

"One naturally thinks that the loss of elements from a system must lead to its degradation, but," Dawkins reasoned, "this is not necessarily so if the elimination is non-random. A sculptor changes a homogeneous rock into a complex statue by subtraction, not addition, of material." In like manner, the shaping of the memory and personality might *require* the discarding of substance not essential to the design!

Dawkins went on to spell out the logic of his fascinating idea. But his article drew a response from Comfort, who believes the concept of the daily demise of brain cells in multimillenary quantities must be put in the category of "neuromythology," inasmuch as the original extrapolations had been made from relatively skimpy data. Moreover, other laboratories had often failed to corroborate the findings. (At Johns Hopkins, for example, Bruce W. Konigsmark and Edmond A. Murphy counted small brainstem samples from twenty-three autopsied cases, ranging in age from newborn to ninety years, and could find no neuronal loss with age in that particular area of the brainstem—though they readily admitted that losses might occur elsewhere.) Echoing Comfort's sentiments was Joseph Tomasch of Iran's Pahlavi University at Shiraz, whose own studies had failed to identify brain-cell deaths in anything like the claimed quantities.

Harold Brody himself, the man whose early studies are among those most often cited as evidence of hourly neuronal hecatombs, never put forth any such specific figure as 100,000 cells a day; nor did he ever profess that his findings—carried out in several areas (though, all taken together, only a small fraction) of the cerebral cortex—necessarily constituted evidence of a brainwide phenomenon. He feels today, as many gerontologists seem to, that neuron death occurs at varying rates in different parts of the aging brain, ranging all the way from near zero in some areas to very large quantities in others, some of them probably critical to the organism's overall function.

At any rate, it is generally assumed that the brain does lose cells, in regions of vital importance, at a rate rapid enough to warrant concern—and that such dead cells are probably not resurrectable. Hence one easily imagines a rejuvenated body with an irreversibly deteriorated brain, a horribly ironic joke to contemplate. Francis Otto Schmidt of MIT once suggested that brain cells might be taught to replace themselves by renewed division, just as the body's mitotic cells naturally do. But even if this were to become feasible, a number of gerontologists—Strehler among them—believe that renewed division of neurons might well result in the destruction of personality and of the individual's sense of identity and continuity, a cruel joke of another sort. What would be the fun of attaining great longevity if the lucky winner couldn't remember what had gone before? If one assumes that personal history—all memory, learning, and experience —is somehow stored in the molecular lattices of our neurons, then renewed mitosis would be expected to break up those patterns, shatter the individual historical record, and thus destroy identity.

One possible route to a longer-lasting brain record, and hence a more durable identity for future generations (though it offers no consolation to anyone already here) would be to start out in life with a larger brain. "One cannot forget," as John Tyler Bonner comments in a *Scientific American* book review, "how different from all other animals man really is, and how all these differences seem to be associated with the extraordinary tumor-like growth of the brain starting only a few million years ago." Many students of human evolution have expressed amazement at this explosive enlargement of the brain—some think as much as a 50 per cent increase in size since *Pithecanthropus* only a half million years ago. There is no reason to consider the current brain as a forever-finished product, as large as it ever will be. Even if its growth were to continue, however, a rate that is deemed "explosive" or "tumor-like" on a geological time scale can be invisibly slow in terms of an individual human lifetime. And evolutionary development, by its very definition, operates in species over many generations, not in any single person's life span.

The always imaginative French biologist Jean Rostand has suggested that all it would take in the course of development would be one additional division of the neurons to double the size of the brain. If we could achieve this by deliberate genetic manipulation—postpone the turning off of the mitotic switches one division longer—we could presumably do it selectively, doubling the number of neurons in some regions (e.g., the cortex) while permitting other regions (e.g., the brainstem) to turn off on schedule. If this had to be done *in utero,* the fetus would be faced with the problem of how to get out, with a head so big. A Caesarian section might be one answer. Or, as Rostand further suggests, if the embryo-fetus-infant were to be developed *in vitro,* a potentially feasible engineering feat, the chamber opening could be made as large as necessary for a comfortable exit. On the other hand, the brain does continue to grow after birth, and it is conceivable that, if neurons need to double again only in limited critical areas of the cortex, such growth might still be contained within the existing cranium.

All this is much more in the realm of fancy, as far as we can presently judge, than some of the possibilities discussed earlier. Moreover, even if it suddenly became practical to carry out Rostand's fantasy, the dilemma posed by dying brain cells would only be postponed, not solved. Might there ever be a way to imprint upon *new* brain cells the patterns that existed earlier? This eventuality has been discussed in speculations about the cloning of new individuals from mature single cells. Though a "clonee" would be an identical genetic twin of the person from whom the cell was taken, he would have a new brain and hence develop a totally different personality shaped by environment and experience. A clonee of an Einstein cell would not be likely to have thought of the theory of relativity, nor an artificial twin of Michelangelo to cope with the Sistine ceiling. So a person of wealth or eminence who wanted to clone himself and produce a reasonable replica of his own individual temperament and talents would be frustrated by this limitation. But would he, necessarily?

Not necessarily, says Strehler. He has designed an elaborate machine (not yet built, but under development) by which he believes a person's essential personality patterns and memories could conceivably be recorded, stored, and imparted to a new brain. Looking over his as yet unpublished plans and patent applications, I am tempted to think of his device—too complex to explain here even if I had his permission, and even if I properly understood it—as a kind of supercomputer. But it is not a computer at all, rather a new invention, a series of interlocking data-processing devices capable of recognizing patterns of information whose importance is reflected by their redundancy, and possessing unprecedented capabilities of storage, manipulation, retrieval, and readout.

I have sat and stood and paced with Strehler literally for hours at a time as he freely discussed his machine. He has patiently explained the gadgetry and the theories which support it. He has produced microphotographs of layered brain tissue, has drawn circuit diagrams, and done a lot of hand-sculpturing in the air to emphasize his points. Drawing from neurobiology, electronics, cybernetics, molecular genetics, information theory, and solid-state physics, he has dazzled me with expositions of how information is handled by the nervous system, in what ways it is analogous to molecular-genetic coder-decoder systems, which layers of neurons perform what kind of function, in what ways his theories and models depart from earlier assumptions. Each time I have almost begun to believe I understood. But later, looking over my notes and his doodles, and searching my own flawed memory, I would finally not be able to put the pieces together again. Yet, somehow, I was convinced that his idea was sound, and that his machine just might work. If the apparatus does perform as Strehler hopes, one could transfer, not all the details, certainly, but the essential patterns from an old brain to a new one that would enable the transferred identity to recognize itself as the same person! If he is right, then even the brain barrier may finally be overcome. (If Strehler can work out so ingenious a machine so early in the game, surely he and others can do better later.)

Meanwhile, though the living brain grows senile, the exploratory study of what makes it age is only in its infancy. As the investigation continues apace, we may entertain a reasonable certainty that new understanding will suggest new ways—now unforeseeable in their specifics—to forestall or slow the rate of neuronal death and central nervous system degeneration. We may hope that, by the time the gerontologists have devised effective means for slowing the body's aging, the neuro-gerontologists will have done as well by the brain.

There of course remain many other barriers to overcome before we need face this "last barrier" which the death of irreplaceable neurons represents.

Chapter XVII

A FRONTIER
IN FLUX

One formidable barrier on the road to a proper scientific understanding of—and thereby perhaps the abolition of—old age is not biological but rather psychological in nature. I am talking, once more, about the credibility barrier. To help overcome it, I have given myself license to go beyond mere reporting. The aging-research picture I have thus presented is perhaps more coherent than most gerontologists see it. This is not to suggest that I have deliberately exaggerated, distorted, or in any way conveyed a fraudulent view of the state of gerontological research today; only that my view—though carefully and honestly arrived at through extensive reading, visiting, and interviewing—does not necessarily reflect the consensual view of gerontology itself. Indeed, no such consensus exists.

I am aware that entire areas of conventional, old-fashioned gerontology have been given short shrift in order to allow a fuller account of some of the more recent avant garde developments. Not that there was a measuring out of words or pages in accordance with some preconceived grand design. I simply let the people and the events unfold as the narrative scheme developed in its own organic fashion. The result is a far from perfectly balanced story. But that would in any case be impossible at this stage of gerontological progress, when what might represent a balanced view to one authority would seem a gross distortion to another. It would have been futile to hope that I might please all gerontologists and slight none; in fact, to slight none would automatically displease others.

Each sortie into the frontier areas of aging research provides a reminder of how totally in flux those frontiers are. While in Boston to attend a meeting not long ago, I took advantage of the opportunity to make a couple of last-minute calls on some gerontological sources. I wanted especially to touch base with F. Marott Sinex of Boston University, whom I had not seen in some time. I enjoy his sharp, skeptical mind, and I wanted to test a few of my evaluations against it. I was also curious to know his own current thinking. I was, moreover, a bit uneasy about how little mention I had thus far made of his work, despite the fact that he is one of the central figures in gerontology today.

One problem, from a storyteller's viewpoint, is that Sinex has not developed any theory of his own, nor does he subscribe to any of the existing theories. "I hate theories," he readily admits, tilting his chair back against the wall, his hands behind his head, grinning his wide sudden grin. "I hate to talk about theories, and I wish other people wouldn't be so fond of them either, especially in a science no more advanced than gerontology is right now. There are lots of observations, lots of ideas, but nothing we should yet dignify with the designation 'theory.'" He nevertheless tolerates, with good humor, my own discussion of various theories.

At the mention of the somatic-mutation theory, whose popularity I have discerned to be on the wane, Sinex says, "Don't rule it out yet. New things are happening. I'm not at all sure I'm not a proponent of it myself—depending on how you describe it." So saying, he bids his secretary furnish me a copy of the chapter he has just finished writing for *The Handbook of Aging*. "Read this and you'll see what I mean."

Discussing prospects for NIH's new Institute on Aging, and speculating as to who might be chosen its director*, Sinex reflects that Hayflick might be a good candidate—one he could certainly approve personally, at any rate, though he doubts that Hayflick could afford to take the job. Just a few minutes later, he is being rather critical of Hayflick's experiments and theories. "If you think he's so wrong," I ask, "why do you consider him qualified to be director of the institute?"

"I didn't say he was *wrong*," he replies, with a quick grin. "I just think some of the interpretations of his work are unwarranted at this stage of the game. That has nothing to do with my opinion of how good a director he'd make."

* The man finally chosen for the job, early in 1976, is Robert N. Butler—a leading authority on the psychology and sociology of aging.

If Sinex isn't on Hayflick's side, theoretically speaking, how does he feel about Denckla? Denckla, I know, has been a recent visiting lecturer at Boston University. "Well, Donner is a very interesting fellow," he comments, cautiously. "He has a lot of fascinating ideas, but we have to reserve judgment. Too much remains to be proven."

Throughout our conversation, Sinex delights in coming up with bits of information—and people—I know little or nothing about, in spite of the quantity of research I have done; and he only pretends to be scandalized (or perhaps only half pretends) at each omission. What—I haven't read Macfarlane Burnet's 1974 book, *Intrinsic Mutagenesis?* What—I haven't heard of Dick Cutler at Baylor, who's been working on RNA transcription as it relates to aging? What— I'm not familiar with the investigation of the repair capabilities of DNA being carried out by Ron Hart at Ohio State?

At one point, in discussing the free radical theory of aging, Sinex asks if I have adequately considered that auto-oxidation of membranes is quite a different phenomenon from the action of what he calls "superoxides"—or that antioxidant activity is not to be confused with the behavior of the natural scavengers of free radicals. I am forced to admit that I really am not aware of these distinctions. He tsk-tsks at me and asks if I don't know the work of Irv Fridovich at Duke University on superoxides. To my distress, I do not. Though I have read everything I could get my hands on by the proponents of the free radical theory, including Denham Harman, Paul Gordon, Richard Passwater, Lester Packer, and A. L. Tappel, and have talked to many gerontologists about free radicals and antioxidants, I cannot recall any mention of Fridovich or superoxides. "Well, those fellows are just behind the times, I guess," says Sinex. What to do? Back to Square One and start over again?

Pondering our conversation, I leave Sinex's office and head for the Boston Biomedical Research Institute to see what D. Rao Sanadi is up to. He is best known for his work on the effects of aging on mitochondria, the organelles that serve as the cell's energy machines. Sanadi, too, tells me of things I haven't heard about elsewhere, such as the work of other researchers at his own institute—Peter Davison, at work on collagen, and Barbara Wright, who is studying the difference between early differentiation and the genetics of aging, using the slime mold as a research model.

Sanadi himself has been working on the flight muscles of the blowfly. Because of the energy required from these cells, fully half their substance is made up of mitochondria. These blowfly mitochondria, as they age, fill up with glycogen deposits, which "have no business being there," but Sanadi has not yet figured out what this means in terms of aging.

Most of Sanadi's work to date, however, has centered on the aging rate of rat-heart mitochondria. He has been able to show that the slowing down of oxidation—or, as one might call it, respiration—in heart mitochondria takes place at roughly the same rate as the decline in functional capacity of the organ itself: perhaps 30 per cent in rats of a given age. Not content with studying heart cells in culture, or isolated mitochondria, Sanadi has also carried out experiments with the entire rat heart, suffusing it artificially with blood so that it continues to beat, though outside any living organism. In these circumstances, he can accurately measure the decline in functional capacity of the whole organ—and, at the same time, isolate the mitochondria and measure the decline of their oxidation, thus attaining a convincing degree of correlation.

Through these studies Sanadi has ascertained that in heart failure, when blood is denied the heart muscle, the mitochondria swell up in a very few minutes. It is mitochondrial malfunction more than anything else that destroys the heart tissue. He is now working on ways to combat this kind of damage.

At the moment of my visit, Sanadi is getting ready to launch several separate projects employing nematodes, especially the species called *C. elegans*. They are so tiny, I must shake the flask and get them in motion before I can make them out—barely—with my unaided eye. Sanadi has several reasons for choosing *C. elegans*. For one thing, it is not a pathogenic species. For another, it has a convenient life span of twenty-five days. Because it is free-living, it can be cultured like bacteria; Sanadi has already worked out methods for boosting its yield by tenfold. It thus becomes a very convenient experimental animal. There is yet another advantage of *C. elegans* over other nematode species: it had only six chromosomes, and they have already begun to be mapped, so that any genetic differences with aging can be more readily pinpointed.

Before I leave his lab, Sanadi describes what seems to me an outlandish experiment he is contemplating carrying out with the nonvolunteer assistance of *C. elegans*. He will take separate batches of the nematodes and treat them with powerful mutagens—chemicals that cause mutations. Undoubtedly, large quantities of the tiny worms will be injured or killed by such treatment. Yet, every now and then there will occur a favorable mutation; so good things are certain to happen to at least some of the survivors. What Sanadi will be looking for is a mutant strain that will suddenly live much longer. Suppose, for instance, that a strain of mutated *C. elegans* were suddenly to live for fifty days instead of twenty-five. The mutation would have doubled the life span. If Sanadi can then ascertain that the mutant strain can transmit its extended life span to its offspring, that will be time enough to start checking out the genetics of this revolutionary evolutionary event and perhaps make some discoveries about the genetics of aging. Some of the discoveries might to some degree be transferrable to the elucidation of human aging.

All this from two casual drop-in visits one morning in Boston.

Very shortly after that trip, I had occasion to drive from Houston to Galveston with Donner Denckla. He too had new data to report, though not yet publishable. Over the next couple of weeks David Harrison came down from Bar Harbor to visit, as did Strehler from California. Both of them updated me on their work and constantly evolving thoughts (Harrison, for example, is reconsidering his assessment of Hayflick). Strehler was in New York to attend a conference on the neurobiology of aging at New York University— which I also attended. And the conference, too, was full of new information and insights. As one example, Harold Brody of SUNY/ Buffalo discussed the notorious "aging" pigment, lipofuscin, the undisposed-of garbage that accumulates in aging nerve cells. He noted that, in some parts of the brain where the cells contain large deposits of lipofuscin, the number of cells remains fairly constant throughout life; whereas in other areas with little lipofuscin, cell deaths are much more numerous! This led someone in the audience to suggest that perhaps lipofuscin was *good* for cells. "Maybe we've been wrong about it all along. Wouldn't it be fascinating if it turns out that lipofuscin is a substance the cell produces to help it *fight off* the aging process?" It was a notion no one took very seriously. The laughs were hearty. But no one pooh-poohed the idea either, in view of Brody's surprising data.

It is clear that one could go on attending meetings, seeing people, reading, visiting laboratories, updating—and continue to return to the typewriter for further revisions. It is possible (though I doubt it) that at some point one would finally reach the end of one's investigations. But by that time, the author might have aged too greatly to be in possession of his faculties, and all that work would have been wasted.

I am conscious, of course, how much has been left out. I have said all too little, for example, about GRC/Baltimore and all the programs that go on there under the directorship of Nathan Shock. Run for years under the aegis of the National Institute of Child Health and Human Development (which has also administered all of NIH's extramural grants in aging research), GRC will now become the research core of the new National Institute on Aging. In a different kind of aging book, GRC/Baltimore might deserve to be at Stage Center most of the time. I have never gone to visit the aging centers at Duke or the University of Michigan. (Their work seems more psychosocial than biological.) At USC's busy gerontology center, I have seen only Strehler and Finch. There are all kinds of tidbits of gerontological data which, though less than worldshaking, have a real interest and charm of their own* and which I would have liked to find room for, but they simply didn't fall naturally anywhere in the framework of my narrative.

I have many technical papers from Germany in German and from Russia in Russian that I have not taken the time to have properly translated. Though I have touched on research in many nations, a number of other nations have gone unmentioned. For instance, I have not come across any reference to gerontological research in Sweden, yet I know there must be good work going on in that scientifically sophisticated nation. But there is no point or profit in feeling guilty about not knowing everything.

I find it less easy to brush aside guilt feelings in regard to the relatively scant attention given to some of the mavericks of aging research. One such is Benjamin Frank of New York. Though I have mentioned him here and there, I have not attempted to explain his theories or his experiments in any fully detailed way. Ben Frank came to me many years ago, when I was science editor at *Life,* hoping that I might do a story about his work and theories. At the time, he was mainly concerned with nutrition and energy; his central idea was that the organism could be energized far beyond the

* One example is a study of the correlation of fingernail growth with age which William B. Bean started—as a purely peripheral interest, in the midst of an extraordinarily busy life, using his own fingernail parings—many years ago in Iowa and continues at UTMB/Galveston, where he is director of its Institute for the Medical Humanities.

"normal" by supplying it dietarily, in single meals, with nucleic acids, proteins, enzymes, and vitamins—giving the cells everything they needed for protein manufacture all at once, including the protein-making machinery in the proper molecular form. Later, it seemed to Frank that such a diet should have anti-cancer and anti-aging effects as well; and, according to his own account, his experimental results to date indicate that his original hunches were correct. Patients placed on his diet not only have more pep, he says, but are *visibly* younger after a period of time. Frank recently added high doses (up to 10 milligrams) of magnesium glycerophosphates to the diet of a few patients, on the theory that, as precursors to substances that are important to the proper function of receptor sites at cell membranes, they should help counteract the effects of aging. (One of his research maxims is: When you want to produce an effect, never give a final product; always give precursors. The final product, he believes, helps only briefly and keeps the body from making its own at earlier stages.) In any case, the phosphate eaters claim—among other benefits—easily detectable improvements in skin condition, including the filling out of wrinkles and the deep grooves around the mouth.

One problem in regard to Ben Frank, whose M.D. degree is from a Swiss medical school, is that he is not and never has been affiliated with any recognized research institution, though he was able to work for a while at Portugal's Gulbenkian Institute, and he has done only small-scale experiments with animals, usually in his own home or office. Moreover, none of his papers has been accepted for publication in journals of established reputation. Though he has written a book—*Nucleic Acid Therapy in Aging and Degenerative Disease*—it is little known and his results have not been adequately tested elsewhere. Hence, he is not recognized by anyone in the biomedical establishment and remains outside the mainstream.

In terms of aging, Frank—like Harman, Sanadi, and others—places great importance on the mitochondria, and especially the whole process of oxidative phosphorylation, the chemical energy cycle that powers the cell. He feels that a few key substances are vital here, one being cytochrome Q, the other NADH. He has worked out his theory in rather great detail, and, while it makes logical sense to me, I lack the expertise to evaluate it. Trying to assess even work done in major institutions by recognized investigators with their published work to draw on, and other experts who are familiar with their work to call upon, is difficult enough. Nevertheless, I feel uneasy about loners like Ben Frank, whom I wish could be given a better hearing.

Then there is Benjamin Schloss, brilliant, vocal, opinionated, a familiar face and voice at gerontology meetings, known but not taken more than half-seriously. He too is very much a lone operator, though he is constantly trying to organize international research programs. He is not affiliated with any institution and has not published widely in first-rate journals. He is a Ph.D., not an M.D., and he is more engineer than biologist. He, too, came to me many years ago, while I was at *Life*. As in the case of Ben Frank, it was difficult to know what to do with him, journalistically. He was originally sent to me by Stanley Kubrick. Schloss got in touch with Kubrick to see if he could interest him in making a movie about aging. Kubrick was preoccupied with other commitments at the time and sent him along to me.

Ben, at the time, was director of something called the Foundation for Aging Research in Brooklyn. I don't know that it consisted of much more than a letterhead, though it had some distinguished names on it. He was largely a propagandist for aging research rather than a researcher himself, though he had worked out a number of theories, most of them dealing with aging as a nuclear genetic program, in the same vein as Strehler and Hayflick. He was impatient to have me do a large story on aging research, but I was not ready; though I had accumulated a couple of drawersful of material, it had not yet fallen into any manageable pattern. For a brief period, Schloss was able to get a grant from the Dreyfus Medical Foundation to work on nematodes—not Sanadi's tiny *C. elegans,* but the larger nematodes which the Gershons had made famous with their work in Israel and which Rothstein was pursuing at SUNY/Buffalo. Schloss worked in Rothstein's lab for a time. When his grant ran out without his having achieved any definitive results, he moved out to Los Angeles where he now lives as a kind of free-lance gerontologist.

Schloss has worked out an elaborate theory of aging that starts with the basic motion patterns of the universe, then works its way down to Earth and living systems and how cells age—and how they might be prevented from aging. I have already described a couple of Schloss's machines, and he has recently started something he calls the One Hundred Year Clubs in Los Angeles; its members aim, by taking the best possible care of themselves, to live to one hundred in the best of health. Ben sees no good reason, however, why we need stop at one hundred—or at any limit.

There are many other mavericks I have not written about—e.g., the cellular therapists of Switzerland (especially the successors of the late Paul Niehans), the various rejuvenators—but these are less on my conscience. For one thing, I have had little personal contact with them and hence feel less responsibility. For another, they have been written about extensively.

I repeat once more what this book has been about up to this point. It has been an exploration of the theories and evidence which have been put forth to suggest that human biomedical science may feasibly hope to make old age obsolete—or at least to postpone it considerably and lessen its ravages—as well as to extend the maximum human life span. The question was: Can we do it? And the answer is: Quite probably, yes, we can.

Chapter XVIII

WHAT YOU MIGHT HOPE FOR PERSONALLY

Before we tackle the more cosmic questions in terms of consequences for the future of humankind, a pause for some practical, personal considerations. Let us assume that gerontological research does hold out a valid promise of additional good years of life. In that case, each of us is bound to wonder whether the hoped-for advances will occur in time to add good years to our own lives—and to the lives of those we wish to share ours with; and, further, what we might meanwhile do to enhance the probability that we will still be on hand to take advantage of whatever breakthroughs may occur.

As I emphasized in Chapter XIV, it is impossible to set forth a precise timetable of upcoming gerontological achievements with any assurance that these events will occur on schedule. This is true even for a given theory or a given investigator. Suppose, as one example, that Donner Denckla succeeds in his quest for the thyroid-blocking hormone, and it turns out to be *the* death hormone, as theorized. How long would it take for the results to start doing us any good? Denckla has recently made some careful calculations, considering each painstaking step along the way: isolating and purifying the hormone (if indeed only one hormone is involved), discovering its structure, synthesizing it, devising some molecular means to inhibit its action; perhaps identifying its releasing factor in the hypothalamus —the smaller molecule that induces the pituitary to release the larger one—and going through the same sequence of procedures with it; getting a sufficient supply of the inhibiting agent to test it on animals; carrying out the necessary animal trials; then—with Food & Drug Administration approval and the informed consent of the subjects

—conducting some preliminary human experiments, followed by broader and more conclusive human trials; and finally getting the new drug on the market. Denckla figures that, even with good luck, going at his present maximum pace it will take him forty years to complete the work. With stepped-up funding and expanded facilities, he feels he might do it in twenty. Thus it is not preposterous for Denckla, who is now only forty, to maintain a reasonable hope that he could become a direct beneficiary of his own research.

Most gerontologists doubt that substantial advances will be made within their own lifetimes. But many do not share this skepticism, and they encourage a cautious optimism in others. Modest progress —much more modest than that envisioned as the finale of Denckla's overall program—might still offer a slowed-down rate of deterioration, enhanced vigor and enjoyment in the later years, some alleviation or even reversal of overt aging symptoms—in a word, a significant postponement of old age as it is customarily experienced (and feared in advance). Human beings who are very young today may hope that, if they remain in reasonably good health through, say, their middle years, they may become the first people in history to have their life spans extended by artificial means—by how many years, no one can say. Gerontologists such as Comfort and Strehler have held out a long-shot hope that, if you can hang on a little longer, and then a little longer, perhaps helped in each case by some of the smaller breakthrough events, it is just barely possible you could still be here and a candidate for further prolongevity when the larger breakthroughs arrive.

The pace of progress in gerontology should quicken as the National Institute on Aging begins to support programs on a broader scale. Within the next decade or so, I believe we will see the proving out of some of the potential anti-aging substances described in Chapter X as well as others yet to be discovered. At least a few should prove to be effective, with acceptably minimal side effects.

A number of antioxidants are already at hand, and some are safely ingestable—among them Vitamin E. Vitamin C* is also an

---

* Vitamin C research seems destined to be controversial for some time to come, in aging as in other areas. In 1949, for instance, a study by H. D. Chope and L. Breslow of the California Department of Public Health indicated that people who tended to live longer had higher-than-average concentrations of Vitamin C in their blood. But their sample was too small to be conclusive. Moreover, Harman fed his mice (the same breed that did live

antioxidant, though less so; and it is supposed to amplify the effects of Vitamin E. A much more powerful antioxidant than either is the element selenium. Traces of it are present in many of our foods, and perhaps we already get all of it that we need—or is good for us. More is not necessarily better. But "supernutrition," as Richard Passwater calls it, the administration of unusually large doses of vitamins and minerals, is a popular trend among biological investigators, and some purely dietary aids to age resistance may well be developed. Selenium will undoubtedly be among the substances studied for that purpose.

The usefulness of antioxidants will depend on the validity of the free radical theory of aging. This does not mean free radicals will have to be shown to be *the* cause of aging, only that they represent an important factor in wear-and-tear damage. We have at least indirect proof that this is so. As Richard Hochschild* reminds us, "Animal studies show that deficiency of vitamin E in the diet leads to damage of exactly the kind predicted. Age pigments pile up faster. Mitochondria, the power houses of the cell, swell and eventually disintegrate, knocking out the energy generating ability of the cell. And lysosomes break open, releasing their digestive chemicals to digest the entire cell. Thus a small amount of free radical damage is multiplied into a devastating sequence of pathological events."

Much of this damage is prevented or repaired by the body's own self-protective mechanisms as well as by antioxidants naturally present. But, as the studies cited by Hochschild—including those of A. L. Tappel—indicate, an antioxidant deficiency clearly reveals extensive free radical damage. When there is such a clear-cut deficiency, antioxidant therapy can definitely reverse the damaging trend. Moreover, substituting one equally effective antioxidant for another will accomplish the same result, proving that it *is* the antioxidant function at work.

Should you therefore begin taking Vitamin E and other antioxi-

---

* Hochschild, working with Strehler at the time, was among those lobbying hard for a National Institute on Aging a few years back. Though the effort failed at the time, and has been largely forgotten in favor of more recent and more successful attempts, the National Institute on Aging would probably not now be in existence except for these earlier sorties into the bio-political arena.

---

longer on other antioxidants) Vitamin C, and it seemed to have *no* life-prolonging effects.

dants? Many people do, including some gerontologists—but the latter have large reservations about taking Vitamin E in the massive doses often recommended. The fact that Vitamin E will counter a specific antioxidant deficiency is not proof—again—that more is necessarily better. Some feel that, with so much still unknown about the precise actions of Vitamin E, there could be some hazard involved. For instance, suppose we were to prevent *too many* of the cell's oxidation reactions; it might impair the cell's functioning in some vital way. So I would recommend caution until such time as more conclusive experiments have been carried out. (In case you're curious, I take 100 units of Vitamin E a day myself, on the grounds that, like chicken soup, it isn't likely to do any harm.)

I do feel optimistic, however, about the potential use of antioxidants in aging, and, because investigators like Harman and Comfort believe the definitive research could be carried out in reasonably short order if sufficiently funded, I include antioxidants as being among drugs probably available in the next decade.

Other good bets for such availability are hormone preparations (such as thymosin), lipofuscin inhibitors (such as centrophenoxine), and lysosome membrane stabilizers (such as the DMAE with which Hochschild has been getting such encouraging results). The same is true of cross-link inhibitors. Robert Kohn, for example, has—in collaboration with F. S. LaBella of the University of Manitoba—had some success with a substance called beta-aminoproprionitrile. Kohn has investigated other possibilities, too, as has Johan Bjorksten. Even though the prevention or reversal of cross-linkages may (like antioxidant therapy to combat free radical damage within cells) fail to get at the basic cause of aging, such an outcome could still prolong the good years of life through "symptom relief." If a drug were to appear that could do no more than uncross-link collagen molecules in the connective tissue outside the cells, the benefits could be considerable.

Collagen, after all, makes up some 30 to 40 per cent of the body's protein. Its universal presence in the body's framework is what has led scientists of Kohn's stature to suggest that the aging of collagen could be a primary factor in the overall aging of the organism. Nutrients going from the bloodstream to the cells must pass through collagen in order to get there. The same is true of waste materials going in the other direction. If collagen becomes dense and rigid, it also becomes less permeable (perhaps even impassable in some cases); hence the cells have a harder time getting their food and getting rid of their wastes, and heart and lungs probably have to work correspondingly harder. Changed collagen molecules could also invite autoimmune attack.

So it is clear that the loosening up of collagen via uncross-linking (or preventing cross-linkage in the first place) could help keep the body younger longer. This would probably be true of appearance as well, since much of the skin's aging and wrinkling could be due to collagen changes. It is even conceivable, as Hochschild further suggests, that it could slow down the graying and falling out of hair. The next decade could be an exciting one, then, in terms of the first visible steps toward anti-aging medications.

Many substances under investigation, such as the temperature-lowering agents of Rosenberg and Kemeny, will undoubtedly take much longer to test because so much is still unknown about the effects of chronic cooling on living organisms. But it is possible that, within two decades, we would know whether such medications are feasible or not—and, if they are, we should by then also have a good idea when we might expect our physicians to be able to prescribe them for us. During this same twenty-year period I think we will also be getting close to arriving at some effective enzyme mixtures and other compounds that would supply substances that were running short and counteract substances that were in damaging oversupply.

During this next twenty or thirty years, a multitude of lines of investigation will be followed simultaneously, and surely some of them will bear fruit. Work such as Denckla's, as we have seen, is problematical, depending on good luck and adequate funding. But I am more optimistic than most about seeing significant progress in hormonal research, in understanding the hypothalamo-pituitary role in aging, in understanding and controlling the on-off switching of genes, and in the general area of genetic engineering. I will venture to predict that by the year 2025—if research proceeds at reasonable speed—most of the major mysteries of the aging process will have been solved, and the solutions adopted as part of conventional biomedical knowledge; and that some of the solutions will by then already have come into practical use to stave off the ravages of senescence.

So you are ready to do whatever is possible to enhance your

chances of being around to enjoy the benefits personally? I'm afraid that the only advice I can offer at this point is the same old-fashioned advice you have always received from your family doctor: Take good care of yourself.

This is always easier to say than to do. Nor is there anything like universal agreement as to what constitutes taking good care of yourself. Even such factors as diet and exercise are controversial—though Alexander Leaf, the investigator who has studied most closely those celebrated pockets of longevity in Ecuador, Hunza, and Soviet Georgia, was able to pin down only two common factors (as reported in his *Youth in Old Age*): all those old folks eat frugally (though nutritiously) and continue to exercise and work hard.

Whole books,* indeed whole shelves full of books have been written, on how to take care of yourself. They are not, needless to say, in total agreement. But it is possible to list some general points I have noted in many years of reading, and of talking with members of the various biomedical professions.

In the realm of diet, the best advice is: Eat lightly. Obviously, even very old people still require a well-balanced and nutritious diet, but the quantity does not have to be large. Obesity is a handicap, especially as you grow older. With your strength diminishing, your heart and lung capacity declining, and your blood-vessel spaces narrowing, you don't need to carry around any extra weight to add to the burdens of your cardiovascular and respiratory systems—to say nothing of the extra tissue that also needs oxygen and nourishment and adds an additional burden to the same overworked systems. So go easy on calories.

Go easy on fats too. We have by now all heard the bad news about cholesterol and its probable role in cardiovascular diseases and heart attacks. Cutting down on foods loaded with saturated fats (eggs, fatty beef, fat-rich dairy products) is undoubtedly a good idea. But, considering what aging research has taught us about polyunsaturated fats and their probable role in the production of excess free radicals, I wouldn't feel safe in eating unlimited quantities of those either. My own stance is to be prudent about all fats, not be fanatical about avoiding them entirely but simply to eat them sparingly.

The same is true of sugar. Research results are contradictory and inconclusive, but excess sugar intake may have a role in heart

* E.g., Earl Ubell's *How to Save Your Life*.

troubles and even in the buildup of cholesterol, not to mention lesser adverse effects such as causing tooth decay. We can probably get all the sugar we need by eating fruits, preferably fresh fruits.

In sum, we don't need a *lot* of any kind of food (except in special cases where the doctor advises otherwise for specific conditions). We should eat well-balanced diets, including at least the recommended daily minimum quantities of vitamins. Fish and seafood provide excellent protein, although some seafood, such as shrimp, is high in cholesterol while low in fat. Poultry is another good source, although it's well to avoid the skin of the chicken or turkey, where a lot of the fat lies. When you eat meat, select the leaner cuts wherever possible. As for dairy products, drink skim milk rather than whole, make your cheese cottage or pot or low-fat whenever you can. Cereals (preferably unsugared) are good for both nutrition and roughage. You can eat bread and other carbohydrates—whole wheat or vitamin-enriched—but not in large quantities; practically all the fresh fruits and vegetables you want, within reason. As for rich desserts—pies, cakes, pastries, ice-cream dishes, and the like— you're better off without them. Try to avoid them, except as an occasional treat.

How you prepare foods is of course important too. Boiled, poached, baked, roasted—almost any other means of cooking is preferable to frying. The typical short-order service of cheeseburger with french fries and apple pie with ice cream is one of the dumbest kinds of meals you can eat, especially if you're getting on in years and have either a high-cholesterol or weight problem.

What of exercise? For most people who do not participate in regular vigorous athletics, it's best to find some congenial way of getting a moderate amount of exercise *regularly*. An occasional spurt of hard exercise or physical work which may be unavoidable, such as the necessity of shoveling snow, or pushing a stalled car, or running to catch a train with a heavy suitcase, can be very dangerous if you haven't been doing anything else for a while. The weekend athlete is a notorious example of someone courting heart trouble. Exercise, if not every day, should occupy a little of your time at least three or four times a week. It should not be so strenuous as to tax you unduly, but strenuous enough to keep you reasonably fit. Here again, books and exercise systems (from aerobics to yoga) abound; almost any of them is better than nothing. In addition to whatever you do at home, you ought to do something outdoors, something fairly easy and enjoyable but preferably something that exercises your whole body: bicycling, swimming, jogging, skating, dancing (this one is mostly indoors, of course), or even just taking long and not-too-leisurely walks. The main point is to move enough to keep your body from becoming stagnant and lethargic. When you're active, your mind works better too. We have placed great emphasis in our society on labor-saving devices, all the way from pushbutton garage doors to golf carts. Saving labor is fine if you're really overworked or just plain worn out. Otherwise it doesn't save a thing. It costs.

Keep moving. Be sensible and moderate about alcohol. Don't smoke. There simply is not a good thing to be said about smoking. If there is a body system it hasn't yet been shown to be bad for, it's because it hasn't been measured yet.

Life style is a difficult thing to define. I guess a principal element, in terms of aging, is how well you can organize your life to deal with stress and challenge—enough to keep you interested and on your toes, but not so much that you can't cope with it.

What of environment? There is not much you can do about it personally, except to avoid undue exposure to environmental hazards and pollution when possible. For everyone's good, refrain from doing anything to add to pollution. Otherwise, act wherever you see the opportunity in clean-up or prevention campaigns.

As for the specific anti-aging possibilities outlined in the early part of the chapter and in previous chapters, keep an eye out for further developments. They will surely appear and be heard—in newspapers and magazines, on radio and television. If you volunteer as an experimental subject for any of these potential remedies, be sure that the consent you give is truly informed.

Finally, you can do your utmost to influence, by whatever means may be at your command, those responsiblbe for biomedical research policy to see that gerontology is adequately encouraged and financed.

That is, if you think it should be.

PART TWO: SHOULD WE DO IT?

"D. Our first question has to do
     with immortality.
 R. Why immortality?
 D. Only because it is the most
     personal matter, literally, that
     can engage the human mind."

                    —Norman Cousins
                     The Celebration of Life

Chapter XIX

THE IMMORTALISTS

Gilgamesh, the legendary king of Uruk, mighty in war and daring in peace, extravagantly endowed with all the juices of life, gave little thought to the prospect that his prodigious energies might one day fail. He had seen death frequently enough, and had not hesitated to inflict it; but, as we might say today, he didn't relate to it personally. Then death took his closest comrade, Enkidu. Gilgamesh was outraged. He wanted Enkidu's company, and he was used to having what he wanted. But this time when he said, They can't do this to me, they could do it to him anyway. He was dismayed at the irrevocability of Enkidu's departure from the world, and now he was haunted by the suspicion that his own everlasting survival wasn't guaranteed either. He grew so obsessed with the fear of death, however far off it might be, that he found no further joy in living. As Ionesco has asked, in our own time, "Why was I born if it wasn't forever?" Or, as Unamuno put it, only a little bit earlier, in *The Tragic Sense of Life,* "If consciousness is . . . nothing more than a flash of light between two eternities of darkness, then there is nothing more execrable than existence."

Gilgamesh was able to shake off his despondency only by resolving that he would live forever. *His* light would last. In his try for immortality, he traveled far to seek out the advice of the most wise, and there was no recipe that he disdained. But finally, understanding that he was human and mortal, he decided to enjoy what he could and accept the inevitable.

The Gilgamesh epic, reconstructed from millennia-old clay tablets, has reverberations for us today. There, as one example, stands

Bernard Strehler, comparing death to Moby Dick and vowing that "We'll get him yet!" Psychiatrist Robert Jay Lifton of Yale, student and chronicler of death in Hiroshima and Vietnam, has evolved a theory which displaces sex (Freud's candidate) as the human psyche's central concern, and substitutes for it death. Lifton believes that the modern individual is torn by his awareness of death, and by his suppression of that awareness; he is oppressed by his mortality, and by his yearning for immortality.* Lifton discerns in each of us "a compelling universal urge to maintain an inner sense of continuous symbolic relationship, over time and space, with the various elements of life . . . a *sense* of immortality . . . a symbolization of his ties with both his biological fellows and his history, past and future."

Tolstoy's Ivan Ilyitch, as he lies dying prematurely of a baffling illness, typifies these contradictory aspects of the human condition. Ivan always "knew" he would have to die (doesn't everyone?); yet, faced with death's imminence, he refuses to accept it—though he finally must. At the same time he wants desperately to go on living, but knows that, where immortality is concerned, the reach for it is as unacceptable as the grasp of it is unattainable.

We need to accept death; but also to accept—and honor—our desire for immortality. Today, the thanatologists are working on one, and the immortalists on the other. Both thanatology and immortalism are products of the new biomedical technology. The immortalist movement is the lesser known of the two, and more to the point of this book. Thanatology operates more within the boundaries of convention.

"As a physician," Jung once said, "I am convinced that it is hygienic to discover in death a goal toward which one can strive; and that shrinking away from it is something unhealthy and abnormal." Jung was, clearly, an early thanatologist.

Even earlier was Plato. As he lay dying, a friend asked him if he could encapsulate, in a single statement, his basic advice for wise living. After a moment's reflection (the story goes), Plato said: "Practice dying." This is the theme of Stanley Keleman's recent

---

* A similar thesis was expounded by Ernest Becker in his brilliant book-length essay, *The Denial of Death,* much admired by Lifton. Joachim E. Meyer of the University of Göttingen, in *Death and Neurosis,* also gives primacy to the fear of death, rating it as much more central in its effects than, say, separation anxiety or the fear of castration.

Living Your Dying, one of dozens of books published during the
past few years on the general subject of death and dying. In one
1974 issue of *The New York Times*'s Sunday book section, eight
such books were included in a single review. The publication ex-
plosion reflects the astonishing growth of the discipline that has
become known as thanatology.

Technology is not neutral. Its solutions give rise to new, usually
nontechnological problems. With the arrival of ever more complex
and sophisticated clinical gadgetry—artificial respirators, kidney-
dialysis apparatus, heart-lung machines, and the like—along with
novel abilities such as the restarting of stopped hearts, and innova-
tive developments such as intensive-care units, it suddenly became
possible to keep dying patients alive (though, in many cases, with
little hope of ultimate rescue) for longer and longer periods of time.
The new capacities raised many bioethical questions: When should
a patient be allowed to "die with dignity"? Who decides—and under
what circumstances may anyone decide—when to "pull the plug,"
when to turn off the "life"-sustaining machinery?

The same new capacities underlined the need for an updated
definition of death. Formerly, when the heart stopped beating, or
the patient no longer breathed, the doctor could safely pronounce
the patient dead. But now those contingencies had become reversible symptoms: cardiac arrest, cessation of respiration. What, then,
could be used as a reliable criterion of death? This was of particular
importance to the transplant surgeon. An organ taken from a
cadaver, if it is to have the best possible chance to work efficiently
in its new host, should be removed as soon after death as possible.
But this time-bound consideration must not cause the coveted
organ—especially if it is a heart—to be excised with unseemly
haste. The surgeon must be certain the corpse is officially and au-
thoritatively non-revivable. "Brain death"—the cessation of the
brain's electrical activity (evidenced by a "flat" electroencephalo-
gram) for an agreed-upon period of time—has now been almost
universally accepted by the medical profession as the certifiable
criterion of irreversibility.

The new preoccupation with the physiological aspects of death,
a preoccupation enforced by medical circumstances, served to focus
renewed attention on its psychological and social aspects as well.
Most students of, and commentators upon, the situation were in
fairly unanimous agreement: we, in this society, are poorly prepared

to face death. In fact, we have practiced something close to a pathological avoidance of the subject in terms of truly coming to grips with the stark reality of our personal demise, be it ultimate or imminent. Moreover, to aggravate the problem, the same biomedical technology that gave rise to the questions about physiological death has also resulted in the psychosocial depersonalization and dehumanization of death. People are increasingly dying in hospitals, attended by monitors and machines instead of by family, friends, and personal physicians.

It is because these truths, once articulated into awareness, seemed so obvious and so pressing that thanatology has spread so rapidly. Seminars and symposia abound. Publications come off the presses in a steady stream. More and more institutions of higher learning have added to their curricula formal courses on Death and Dying—and soon no self-respecting medical or nursing school will be without one. Most people have applauded this movement (I joined in the applause) as being in the direction of health and sanity, and long overdue.* Thanatology has undoubtedly helped many thousands of patients to face their deaths with greater understanding and equanimity, thus also making more bearable the emotional burdens of the bereaved.

But now—encouraged by gerontology—come the immortalists. Their attitude naturally differs sharply from that of the thanatologists, inasmuch as their fond hope is to render thanatology obsolete. They feel that human beings think *too much* about death rather than too little; that we have all been too accepting of death—and that such a viewpoint is self-defeating, serving to perpetuate death. If you believe something is inevitable, they argue, then it surely will be. Immortalists decry the tradition which rates an individual's wisdom by the equanimity with which he faces his death. "It is precisely this orientation to death which hinders us from launching a global crash movement to overcome mortality," writes Iranian-born novelist F. M. Esfandiary (now at the New School for Social Research in New York) in *Up-Wingers: A Futurist Manifesto*. "Humans are still too death-oriented too guilt-ridden too submissive and fatalistic to demand immortality. To even hope for it."

---

* The most active organization in this field is the Foundation of Thanatology, based at Columbia University. Its founder and president is Austin H. Kutscher, a stomatologist (specialist in diseases of the mouth and jaw) at the Columbia-Presbyterian Medical Center in New York City.

There are scientists, such as Strehler, who talk of defeating death. But what they really intend is the further postponement of death, the extension of the human life span beyond (perhaps well beyond) its present limits. But people like Strehler do not qualify as immortalists. Immortalists aim not to die at all.

And when they speak of "immortality," they are not referring to any kind of vicarious immortality such as the creation of works of art that will live on in posterity's esteem, or as memories in the minds and hearts of loved ones. They know that books can be burned, buildings torn down, cities covered with sand; that even pyramids erode away in the fullness of time. Nor are they inspired by the notion that their atoms and molecules will never disappear but will simply keep changing and merging with other universal forms, an idea that brought solace to the likes of Democritus and Lucretius. Not even cloning would do; the creation of new beings identical to themselves biologically, cloned from their own cells, would have no meaning—unless their own personality, identity, and history could be impressed upon the new brain by some means such as the super-computer envisioned by Strehler. Even this would not satisfy some, who will settle for nothing less than personal immortality; an immortality that means, quite literally, eternal life—or at least indefinite life—with the same consciousness aware of itself and its own history through time.*

Alan Harrington, the novelist, sounded the central theme in the opening sentence of *The Immortalist,* published in 1969: "Death is an imposition on the human race, and no longer acceptable." His flyleaf quote was Unamuno's "All or nothing! . . . Eternity, eternity! . . . that is the supreme desire!" By then, Robert Chester Wilson Ettinger had already published *The Prospect of Immortality,* which launched the cryonics movement. Ettinger advocated the freezing of dead bodies rather than their burial or cremation, to preserve them in as intact a condition as possible against the day

* When, in Norman Cousins's imaginary dialogue in *The Celebration of Life,* the Docent asks, ". . . can you conceive of immortality without continuity of personal memory?", the Respondent answers: "No. How can I be expected to contemplate the meaning of immortality if my immortal self would not know who my mortal self was? If I am deprived of continuity of memory, how would I know I was immortal? Obviously, I would have to know later who I am now. And I want to know now that I shall know this later." (Later in the dialogue, the Respondent settles for a lesser—or at least a different—version of immortality.)

when the infinitely more knowledgeable medical science of the future could thaw them back into renewed life. The cryonics movement (its watchword: "Freeze—wait—reanimate") is an integral part of the immortalist movement. Though all cryonicists are immortalists, all immortalists are not necessarily cryonicists. Nevertheless, if the origin of the current immortalist movement can be pinpointed to a single event in time, it was probably the publication of Ettinger's prophetic and evangelistic book.* Despite the bizzare-sounding nature of his proposals, Ettinger writes with intelligence, clarity, and good humor.

A professor of physics at Highland Park College in Michigan, Ettinger worked out much of his thesis during a three-year hospital stay recovering from wounds suffered in the Battle of the Bulge during World War II. He was of course aware how outlandish his fantasy of a freezer-centered society would sound to conventional ears. He also knew that there did not yet exist the cryobiological know-how to freeze even a much simpler organism than a human body without doing further damage in the freezing process itself. As a consequence, a cadaver would not only still be dead on thawing at some later date, but would have undergone further deterioration by virtue of having been frozen—a deterioration perhaps compounded by the unfreezing process as well. Nonetheless, Ettinger was serious about his proposition, and still is. Some day, he reasoned, scientists might be able to revive the dead and repair damage or disease of any nature, since none of it would be irreversible. In fact, depending on the state of the biomedical arts at the time of revival, the cryonic time-traveler might even be rejuvenated in ways that render him healthier than he ever was in his earlier incarnation. Many things could go wrong meanwhile, of course (my wife, for instance, suggests a power failure that would result in a mass premature thawing), and the realistic prospects of renewed life for a corpse now frozen are admittedly remote. But, Ettinger emphasizes, *they are not zero*. Hence the long gamble, in his view, is worth taking. You are dead anyway, he argues, so what have you got to lose?

One thing you might have to lose, of course (not you, but your heirs or next-of-kin), would be money. Freezing requires storage space, and energy, and rental payments. A reviewer of my earlier book, *The Second Genesis: The Coming Control of Life,* in which

---

* Ettinger has since published a follow-up book, *Man Into Superman,* which seeks to delineate a future worth waking up into.

at one point I briefly described the cryonics movement and its aims, commented, in the course of a generally complimentary review: "Rosenfeld may be a bit uncritical at times. He discusses the controversy over freezing corpses, for example, without mentioning the pathetic emotional misery of survivors duped into this grisly racket." I am not up-to-the-moment on the finances of cryonic interment (as of early 1975, the initial costs amounted to some $15,000, with maintenance charges of $1,800 a year; and it was estimated that a $50,000 insurance policy would cover it all), but the dedicated working people in the movement—nearly all of whom work for no pay—respond with indignation to having their project labeled as any sort of "racket." I assume that anyone who is seriously considering being frozen will spend the necessary time looking into the economic details. It is not in any case my intention to sell anyone on being frozen (I personally have no such plans); what I want to emphasize is that Ettinger has struck a sufficiently responsive public chord to give rise to such practical questions.

Cryonics societies exist in several parts of the United States as well as in other countries of the world. For a while, several hundred members of the Life Extension Society (which is now disbanded as a separate entity) carried Medic Alert wristbands and cards with emergency instructions for rushing them, on death, to the nearest available cryonics facilities. Several such facilities do now exist, with names like Manrise, Trans Time, and Cryo-Span, as well as mobile vans equipped for rapid freezing by the latest methods, designed to do the least possible damage and to maintain the corpse in the best possible condition over whatever period of time may turn out to be necessary. The cryonic version of keeping an eternal light burning —liquid nitrogen at 320 degrees below zero (Fahrenheit)—is obviously not a matter to be undertaken lightly.

Cryonics groups have been able to enlist a number of scientific advisers, which suggests that these scientists—though not necessarily cryonicists themselves—are at least open-minded about the long-term possibilities. Most scientists still believe the whole cryonics movement to be nonsense, and some find it downright repugnant. (Medawar, arguing against the Ettinger Way, writes: "There is another still more compelling reason for dismissing any such idea from our minds: the preservation of life in the deep freeze is a gross affront to all sense of the fitness of things.") A few scientists do take it seriously. There are, for instance, Jean Rostand and

Gerald Gruman, who wrote the two prefaces to Ettinger's book. Physicist Gerald Feinberg of Columbia—the man who conceived the hypothetical, faster-than-light particle, the tachyon, and author of *The Prometheus Project*—is both a cryonicist and an immortalist. And one of the most active members of the Australian cryonics movement is the mathematician Thomas Donaldson.

Ettinger's hope is that the movement will help accelerate research in cryobiology, speeding the day when better freezing techniques will be available. If such techniques ever are perfected and accepted, Ettinger envisions the time when people can choose to be frozen before death—someone with terminal cancer, for instance, may want to be frozen until a cure is discovered; or someone bored with this life in this age might want to try his luck in a later era. Benjamin Franklin, who predicted an eventual 1,000-year life span, once expressed the desire to revisit the future. And John Hunter, the great eighteenth-century British anatomist and surgeon, said he would like to be thawed out for a year every hundred years. A multitude of science fiction plots have by now evolved around Ettinger's theories and fantasies.

The first cryonic nonfuneral in real life took place in early 1967. The freezee was James H. Bedford, a professor of psychology in Glendale, California, who died of cancer at the age of seventy-three. He was stored at the required −320°F in a cryo-capsule and shipped to a cryo-crypt facility in Phoenix, Arizona. Late in 1974, the twenty-fourth official freezing took place. This time the dead person was a six-year-old leukemia victim. (Robert Nelson of the Cryonics Society of California participated in both these freezings—though not, of course, all those in between, many of which were carried out in other places.) Though the official count of cryonic interments adds up to not much more than these two dozen,* it is believed that many more have taken place quietly. Persistent though unconfirmed rumors hold, for instance, that Walt Disney was among those frozen without publicity.

At the time of the Bedford freezing, one member of the Life Extension Society was quoted, in *Life,* as remarking: "If my five-year-old asks me, 'How old will I be in 1,000 years?' I answer, 'You'll be 1,005.' " Another member said he was tape-recording his ideas, trying to delineate his personality, temperament, and life history for

* In January 1972, there was a standby alert when Ettinger's wife, Elaine, underwent surgery, but she recovered nicely.

the benefit of future psychiatrists who would presumably be responsible for helping him adjust to the radically different world into which he might be resurrected. (Ettinger has advocated preserving as much information as possible, not for the use of psychiatrists, but rather of neurologists who would use it to replace information lost in damaged parts of the brain. "The time will certainly come," he said, anticipating Strehler, "when the brain's method of coding memories is thoroughly understood, and messages can be 'read' directly from nervous tissue, and also 'read' into it." He has never been keen, however, on the idea of imprinting the old personality on a newly cloned duplicate brain. "I wouldn't pay a nickel to have a twin of me built after my death," he says flatly.)

Updated information on the cryonics movement is available through a number of small publications. The one I happen to get is the newsletter of the Cryonics Society of Michigan, *The Outlook.** edited by Patrick R. Dewey, who is still in his twenties—proving that you don't have to be old to start thinking about postponing death. A surprising number of very young people do.

Some immortalists feel a bit uneasy about being too closely identified with the cryonics movement because, for one thing, immortalism is not dependent upon cryonics, and, for another, they fear that some people who might otherwise be attracted to the immortalist philosophy may be put off by the cryonic idea. Cryonicists themselves certainly do not tout their way of thinking as The One True Path to Immortality; they simply regard it—in the absence of any practical alternative—as the only way that anyone currently dying can hope to win a long-shot gamble on a renewed stretch of life. They hope, of course, that accelerated research in cryobiology will increase the odds. Hence Ettinger's basic advice: "Try to stay alive a little longer."

Thus, even to Ettinger and his followers, cryonic interment is merely a stopgap measure, something to do while waiting for the larger gerontological breakthroughs to occur. They look for the day when it will no longer be necessary to freeze anyone, because no one will sicken incurably, or grow senescent, or die, except by some overwhelming accident which destroys the body beyond hope of retrieval (though what constitutes "beyond hope of retrieval" will also change with time).

* Its name has just been changed to *The Immortalist.*

"Immortality," says Esfandiary in *Optimism One,* "is only another phase in evolution. It is no more spectacular than the evolution of the upright position or the attainment of speech. Certainly it is far less spectacular than the emergence of life from matter." And in *Up-Wingers:* "Immortality is now a question of how and when—not if."

In *Man Against Mortality,* Dean F. Juniper of the University of Reading School of Education in England, sums up: "Life itself is, on the best evidence, not immortal. It is also very clearly not the same thing as inanimate matter, which is slowly simplifying. Life is constantly renewing itself, striving to keep itself going in a world of steady simplification by taking inanimate matter and using it to maintain itself, in a kind of fluctuating battle, the skirmishes of which are births and deaths.

"And it is surely not too fanciful to suggest that if there is a battle, life may eventually triumph—not in the precarious sense in which we see it at present, but in a total, unconditional victory. In this war man may be life's ultimate weapon. *He may be designed to make himself and life immortal, the necessary skills and motivations having been built into him.* [Italics supplied.] If this is the case then all his myths and fantasies of immortality may be in the nature of necessary rehearsals for an as yet unrealistic, but eventually to be realized, ultimate transformation."

Probably the best single source of information about the immortalist movement is A. Stuart Otto, editor of *The Immortality Newsletter,* which he has been publishing monthly from his home base in San Marcos, California, since October of 1970. Otto has made it his mission to gather—and to disseminate as widely as possible—all such information, and has given generous permission for anyone to use any of it for whatever purpose; he copyrights nothing. He appreciates a credit line, but use of the material is unconditional.

Otto is an interesting individual who leads two separate lives—one as A. Stuart Otto, editor of the newsletter, the other as Friend Stuart, official and member of what he describes as "a small Christian metaphysical denomination." Though he holds the equivalent of a doctor of divinity degree, the only title used in his church is "Friend." His books employ a religious rather than a secular approach, "and when I write in that area," he explains, "I do so as Friend Stuart—not as a pseudonym, but because that is my correct professional name in that field." Because *The Immortality Newsletter* is "basically oriented in a scientific direction," he edits it under his secular name, his aim being "to reach individuals who might be turned off by a spiritual approach per se."*

Friend Stuart's own essential immortalist book is *How to Conquer Physical Death*. His thesis, oversimplified, is curiously similar to that of Shaw's Franklyn Barnabas: you achieve continued life by *willing* it. Shaw himself, that supreme rationalist and intellectualizer, seemed in his later years to have developed the belief that evolution may have come about through a kind of intense protoplasmic yearning for it. His creation, Dr. Barnabas, tells the politicians: "Do not mistake mere idle fancies for the tremendous miracle-working force of Will nerved to creation by a conviction of Necessity. . . . They will live three hundred years . . . because the soul deep down in them will know that they must, if the world is to be saved." Friend Stuart does not of course stop at three hundred years. He believes that there might well already exist beings among us who have lived many lifetimes—who are in fact immortals—and who would not be likely to reveal this to the rest of us in the current state of our development. But he believes that the secret, which he purports to reveal to us in his book, is available to any one of us.

It is no wonder that Stuart Otto is attracted to the work of Lawrence Casler, a psychologist at the State University of New York in Geneseo. Casler has begun two basic experiments, one of which will have reasonably early but inconclusive results; the other will have to wait for its dénouement until—well, until what a non-immortalist would have expected to be a time after Casler's life was over. Casler himself is an immortalist and so will not be surprised if he is here to report the results.

His basic method is simple. He uses hypnosis to implant the idea of longevity. First he used a small group of elderly patients, putting aside half of them as a control group. Later he recruited a larger group from among his students, who have promised to keep in touch over the years. The aim is to see if he can implant a real belief in the subject that he will live much longer than the normal life expectancy—say, 120 years; and to see if this belief actually does add years to the subject's life. (A number of orthodox psychologists do believe that emotional attitudes can affect longevity, at least to a limited extent.)

* This publication's title has also been changed very recently to *Theologia 21*, suggesting a departure from earlier policy.

The hard core of immortalists strive for literal immortality—living forever—or at least, as Dean Juniper puts it, "the amount of time that any man might wish to live supposing that he had the power to do so"; thus "a state of absolute choice." But people like Ettinger and Alan Harrington will settle for less. They know eternity is a long time. As Harrington puts it, "What must be eliminated from the human situation is the inevitability of death as a result and natural end of the aging process. I am speaking of the inescapable parabolic arching from birth to death. But we must clearly understand that any given unit of life—my individual existence and yours—can never be guaranteed eternity.

"Until such time as duplications of individual nervous systems can be grown in tissue cultures (at this point no one knows 'whose' consciousness they would have), our special identities will always be subject to being hit by a truck or dying in a plane crash. A sudden virus or heart seizure, even in the body's youth, may carry us off. Statistically, looking ahead thousands of years, the chances are that every human and even inanimate form will be broken sooner or later. But the distress felt by men and women today does not arise from the fear of such hazards. Rather, it comes from the certainty of aging and physical degeneration leading to death. It is the fear of losing our powers and being left alone, or in the hands of indifferent nurses, and knowing that the moment must come when we will not see the people we love any more, and everything will go black. . . .

"In our conception immortality is *being alive now, ungoverned by span, cycle or inevitability.*"*

Harrington discusses various symbolic ways of "defeating" death, but is tough about insisting that "the struggle against real death requires training, and must be fought out industrially and in the laboratory." His faith, unlike Friend Stuart's, is altogether non-metaphysical. "This new faith we must have," he insists, "is that with the technology at our disposal in the near future death can be conquered. . . . Our new faith must accept as gospel that salvation belongs to medical engineering and nothing else; that man's fate depends first on the proper management of his technical proficiency;

---

* In the late eighteenth century, Condorcet had a similar vision of a day "when death will be nothing more than the effect either of extraordinary accidents, or of the slow and gradual decay of the vital powers; and that the duration of the interval between the birth of man and his decay will have itself no assignable limit."

that we can only engineer freedom from death, not pray for it; that our messiahs will be wearing white coats, not in asylums but in chemical and biological laboratories."

Having said and reported this much about immortalism, and conveyed some of its flavor, I now feel obliged to append a reminder that the movement is still small in official membership, and that its scientific proponents are few indeed. But its existence, and the vigor and enthusiasm of its adherents, suggest that many people have strong yearnings in this direction—for longer life, if not for the whole immortalist package ("We don't crave immortality," said Pindar, in the fifth century B.C., "but we must reach out to the limits of what is possible for mankind"). Hence my feeling of certainty that, once the capacities for extending the human life span are at hand, there will be plenty of volunteers for the benefits which so many others still rate as dubious.

Nevertheless, the mere contemplation of a designed immortality raises strong misgivings in the breasts and brains of many thinking, feeling people, who worry about the human consequences of even a fractional gerontological success in extending the life span.

Chapter XX

CONSEQUENCES

In W. W. Jacobs's famous short story, "The Monkey's Paw," an elderly British couple comes into possession of an ancient, shriveled monkey's paw. Its owner, they are told, is entitled to make three wishes. But the previous owner of the paw warns the old man: "It had a spell put on it by an old fakir, a very holy man. He wanted to show that fate ruled people's lives, and that those who interfered with it did so to their sorrow." The old man is properly cautious. He decides to make a safe, modest wish: He wishes for £200. Exactly that sum of money does arrive the next day, but in the form of a compensation payment for the death of their son in a horrible accident. The second and third wishes do nothing to rescue the situation.

There must be few human cultures whose literature and folklore do not contain such cautionary tales. Our most deep-seated Jungian natures seem to harbor large suspicions as to the advisability of tampering with the "natural" order of events, even when we have the opportunity to do so for our own benefit. (*Especially* if we do so for our own benefit.) We are convinced that even the smallest and most innocent request will cost us more than it is worth. It will be misunderstood, misinterpreted, misapplied; it will, somehow, backfire on us. There is always a catch to the gift request. As in the case of Faust—or the owner of Stevenson's Bottle Imp—a pact must be made with the devil, who extracts his implacable due.

In the brash scientific era, our Faustian Western civilization has been cavalier about interfering with the natural order of events, sometimes on an impressive scale. But the consequences—in terms of pollution, overpopulation, ever more destructive weaponry, social and personal stress—seem to confirm our soul-felt fears about the hazards of such tampering. Where medicine is concerned, it does not really surprise us that every medication, every therapy comes with a built-in likelihood of adverse side effects, from mild to lethal. Even those medical measures which have had an undeniably curative or life-prolonging effect—where the benefits plainly outweigh the risks for the ailing individual patient—are not without their controversial aspects. When therapies are discovered that keep alive the victims of various hereditary (or partially hereditary) afflictions, people who would otherwise have died at earlier ages—and keep them alive long enough to marry and have children of their own—we applaud the medical victory. But some geneticists grumble that such practices may have deleterious effects on the human gene pool. When the malarial swamps of a poverty-stricken, heavily peopled area are sprayed with DDT, the mosquitoes are destroyed and countless human lives saved (cheers all around). But the population then spurts rapidly beyond the region's food resources, and soon just as many people are dying of starvation as formerly died of malaria; and who knows in which organs of the area's non-insect inhabitants the DDT may have settled?

Despite such caveats, few people have any real qualms about applying medications, surgery, or any biotechnology that might cure, prevent, or ameliorate the suffering and discomfort of the sick and injured. There is much more hesitation, however, at the prospect of tampering with the human life span, for is it not right that a person should die at his appointed hour? Even gerontologists like to cite the story of Tithonus, out of Greek mythology. Tithonus, prince of Troy, was loved by the goddess Aurora, who persuaded Jupiter to grant him immortality. The bad news was that she forgot to specify youth and strength to go with the added years. Though godlike in his immortality, Tithonus was as subject to senescence as any mortal. He grew old, feeble, utterly miserable, wishing for death but condemned to go on living. It was for him that Tennyson wrote the lines: "And after many a summer dies the swan/Me only cruel immortality/Consumes . . ." (Aurora finally turned Tithonus into a grasshopper, which was, I guess, a solution of sorts.)

Searching for the roots of human despair, Kierkegaard, in *Sickness Unto Death,* virtually equated it with a revulsion against the obviously dismaying—to him—possibility that the individual might be condemned to eternal existence, with no end and no escape. Certainly the eternal wheel of existence in ancient Oriental belief evoked despair in the breasts of millions of the miserable throughout the generations; and the promise of escape from that wheel through the attainment of Nirvana must have been one of the great attractions of Buddhism.

The theme of immortality as a curse is carried on through the centuries, as evidenced, for example, in the eternally senile Struldbrugs encountered by Gulliver on Luggnagg, or more contemporarily, in Robert Silverberg's *A Matter of Life and Death*—or René Barjaval's *The Immortals,* where immortality, conferred by a highly contagious mutated virus, keeps plants eternally in flower so that they can never bear fruit. Gerontologists have no interest, of course, in turning us into a race of Tithonuses or Struldbrugs. What they seek to extend is not the period of senility, but the good vigorous years of life. Whenever people have succeeded in doing this—in literature— what they have achieved is usually made to seem wrong, even sinful. The central character of Karel Čapek's 1925 play, *The Makropoulos Secret,* is a woman who has been able to keep herself alive and relatively young for some 300 years by the use of a secret formula. She has lived several lives under several names. A small group of people who have learned the truth about her gather in a room. One man, Gregor, taking the stance of a prosecuting attorney, intones: "The accused, Emilia Marty, a singer. She is accused before God and us of fraud and falsification of papers for her own selfish purposes. And furthermore and in addition, she has transgressed against all trust and decency—against life itself! That does not belong to human judgment. She will have to answer for it in a higher court."

Such a view may seem extreme to us in the mid-1970's, but I believe it accurately reflects the disquiet people often feel about prolongevity. A few years ago, I participated in the Committee for the Future's first SYNCON (for "synergistic convergence") at Southern Illinois University at Carbondale. SYNCON is a rather complex kind of conference, usually a week long, in which various "task forces"—each with its own "coordinator," each assigned a particular area of human concern—meet in the separate, walled-off rooms of a large, circular structure out of whose hub the leaders operate. The assignment for Carbondale was grandiose by necessity: to set, for the next twenty years, goals and a program by which the human species could move toward solving some of its pressing global problems. During the week, walls were removed here and there so that different task forces in related fields could interact. Toward the end of the week, all the walls came down so that everyone could come together in a large confrontation and sharing. At this time each coordinator was to reveal to the assembled conference the goals his own task force had set; then we would see what kind of consensual program we might arrive at. As coordinator of the biological task force, I was called on early. One of the high-priority goals we had set, I said, was a program directed toward the conquest of old age and the extension of the human life span.

Hands went up all over the place.

The first to speak was a clergyman who was coordinator of one of the other task forces. "I would think," he said firmly, "that extending the human life span would be one of our *lowest*-priority goals—if indeed we should undertake it at all at this time in our history.

"Many of my parishioners," he continued, "are bored with life at forty. I spend a lot of my counseling time trying to give people a reason for getting up the next morning and just making it through the day. Now, until we can make it worth people's while to live for seventy years, it seems pointless to try for a hundred and seventy!"

Applause.

The next person to object was the coordinator of the environmental task force. She, too, thought that an anti-aging program should be last on our list rather than first. Considering the problems of pollution, overpopulation, diminishing resources (indeed much of the SYNCON's attention had been focused on the "Limits to Growth" thesis) that already plagued us, she was horrified that we would even tolerate the idea of keeping people around longer, thus aggravating all our afflictions.

More applause. And other speakers took their turns, voicing one objection after another, ranging all the way from the very personal to the global, cosmic, and evolutionary.

It is clear that the idea of living longer does not win anything like automatic or universal assent. Many people are downright hostile to the idea. The immortalists argue that many harbor negative feelings about longevity out of conditioning and habit, and because they believe they have no choice anyway; but that, if there did exist a real and believable option to live out a longer span of good years, a number would change their minds and vote the other way. I think this is probably true. Nevertheless, I believe a great many individuals —even given the choice—would still choose to let nature bring life to its current culmination. (The assumption, of course, is that no one would be forced to take advantage of the option to live longer.) And their reservations are not merely the unthinking expressions of anti-progressive bias. They rather bespeak a valid concern, deeply felt in both brain and belly, that our most prized human values may be in danger.

"Perhaps the biggest threat to the human race at the moment," wrote Kenneth Boulding in the *Bulletin of the Atomic Scientists* in 1970, "is not so much the nuclear weapon as the possibility of eliminating the aging process.

"If we could rearrange the human genetic structure to program death at the age of 1,000 [thirty-one years older than Methuselah] rather than at 70 . . . the human race would face the biggest crisis of its existence, a crisis which I illustrate easily to an academic audience by asking them who wants to be an assistant professor for 500 years."

Longevity does have consequences. And the consequences, if we were all to live a thousand years, starting tomorrow, would be over-whelming. It is not that Boulding believes anyone is likely to chance upon the kind of breakthrough that would permit individuals now alive to enjoy the millennial life spans of the biblical antediluvians. Gerontological success, when it begins to be achieved, will probably arrive in much more modest increments. In the long run, of course, the problems created by increased longevity will be so far-reaching as to exceed our present ability to imagine them.

Not that we are trying very hard to imagine them. Robert Heil-broner has noted that human beings, despite verbal expressions to the contrary, do not truly care about posterity. They cannot relate to it in a personal way; the individual welfare of their children, yes, or even their grandchildren; but, beyond these limited familial responsibilities, the future (even 50 or 100 years off) is somewhere Out There, too remote to warrant much of today's worry energy. Later generations, with their more highly developed science and technology—we tell ourselves—will surely figure it all out when the time comes. Meanwhile, like Candide and Cunegonde, we must hoe our gardens.

"However altruistic we may be," says Dean Juniper, "we are usually capable of stifling our anxieties about those of our acts whose consequences will affect our descendants. We tend to talk in rather lofty ways about building for the future, but those plans do not carry the flavor of anxiety with them."

Those who have most energetically tried to imagine what human beings might be like if they were to live indefinitely are, as might be expected, the science fiction writers. And their writings do usually carry "the flavor of anxiety" that Juniper finds missing in the rest of us. This anxiety shows through even in the imaginings of fairly optimistic writers like Robert Heinlein, who has succeeded in conjuring up a number of tolerably livable futures. Typical is Alan E. Nurse's story, "The Martyr," in which many of the long-lived characters seem to have a hard time getting anything accomplished. Under the euphoric influence of knowing that they always have plenty of time, there is never any need to hurry. The members of a research team preparing to launch a large space ship seem to be constantly on the verge of completing the project; but then someone sees a way to make the ship, and the mission, a little more perfect and—since there is plenty of time—why not? So they keep tearing everything apart and starting all over again, until it becomes apparent to a newly arrived engineer on the project that they are never going to get the ship launched at all.

Some writers have, in fact, imagined scenarios in which the human race becomes much less adventurous, in which that long stretch of life becomes so precious that its beneficiaries are obsessed with mere survival. Perhaps the ultimate story in this genre is Stephen Leacock's "The Man in the Asbestos Suit," from *Afternoons in Utopia*. Leacock envisions a once-great city, several centuries hence, where no one ever dies of anything but accident or injury. All the inhabitants go about encased in protective asbestos suits, spending all their time being careful, concentrating every attention on not having an accident.

Would longer-lived individuals really lose their sense of adventure, their zest for engaging in risk-taking enterprises? If so, society would stagnate—which it of course could not afford to do. A civilization inhabited by people wholly concerned with their personal survival at all costs would end up defeating their own ends by rendering impossible the survival of the civilization that sustains them; for civilizations require high technology, and the taking of risks to cope with change, in order to sustain themselves. I suppose we might one day arrive at a point where we could turn the whole global enterprise over to a giant computer, though presumably we would still require some human repair, monitoring, and reprogramming capabilities.

If people lived longer, would they really be more easily bored— or less so? Would they be happier, more creative, more "human" (whatever we think that means)? Would we prize our lives, and those of others, more—or less? Would we be readier to go when death ultimately arrived, or would we fight it more bitterly? Would our natures be kinder, or more ruthless? Obviously, our feelings about life and death would—then as now—be individual and conflicting. As the Cambridge philosopher Bernard Williams points out, in *Problems of the Self,* "Death is said by some to not be an evil because it is not the end, and by others, because it is. . . ." Williams himself declares that immortality would be intolerable, but he does concede that it might be nicer to live longer. How much longer? He would elect to die "shortly before the horrors of not doing so became evident." It is likely that much of our character and temperament, our social attitudes and ethical standards, would be heavily dependent upon the overall context in which we lived. And, at any given time in the future, the quality of that context would in turn depend upon how satisfactorily we managed the population problem.

"It has been calculated," writes Juniper in *Man Against Mortality,* "and this gives us an idea of the extraordinary capacity of geometrical increase, that if life had been unnegated from the beginning, that is, if it had not been accompanied by death, we should now be part of a solid ball of flesh expanding into the universe at a speed approaching that of light." And even this, he adds, is "a fantastically qualified speculation." He then goes on to make some scary extrapolations.

It is clear that, if people stay around for longer periods of time instead of dying off on the old schedules, they will fail to make room for new arrivals. Thus, whatever birth ratios make for Zero Population Growth in the 1970's will not hold for the ensuing decades and centuries. People who remained alive and vigorous longer would continue to consume the earth's resources through all those added years, and therefore—based on present technologies— use them up at an accelerated rate. They would also continue to add their wastes and garbage and the emanations of their machines and appliances, thus also accelerating the rate of planetary pollution.

Moreover, inasmuch as we are assuming that the new breed of

long-livers will remain younger, physiologically, for considerably extended periods of time, we may also assume that their reproductive periods will be lengthened, so that couples (or single women) can and may well want to go on having children far beyond the usual cutoff point. Gilbert W. Kliman, director of The Center for Preventive Psychiatry in White Plains, New York, has observed that some women only seem happily secure when they are pregnant; this is, unfortunately, often true of disturbed or retarded women. Though they lose interest in the children once infancy is past, they like to go on having babies. If people were to remarry—an increasing likelihood as lives grow longer—and still had energetic years of life to look forward to, they might choose to have new families with their new spouses.

As time goes on, the probability clearly grows that governments may have to intervene in traditionally sacrosanct personal and familial areas. As Juniper puts it, "we can deduce a strict control of immortalist men and women, in terms of a sophisticated, foolproof, psychopath-proof system of ensuring that the option of immortality also entails sterility." The day might well arrive when would-be parents were required to apply for a license to have a child—and, in order to do so, would have to wait for a vacancy.* (Since they would have a lot of time, they might not mind the wait so much.) Enforcing such a requirement, especially making it as foolproof as Juniper suggests, would of course be fraught with difficulties.

One inherent difficulty is that something positive must be done, as matters now stand, to *prevent* conception. How order people to take that positive step, in an intimate transaction, and see that they comply? Now, if people were *in*fertile under ordinary circumstances and had to take some positive step to render themselves fertile, the situation would become easier to control. Francis Crick of DNA fame has suggested that contraceptive substances (which, by then, would presumably be safe and effective) might be put in the public water supply; then some antidote would have to be administered, the substance perhaps available only on prescription from a licensed practitioner and issued only to an approved parental licensee.

---

* Boulding has more than half seriously suggested a "green stamp" plan, in which each young person in a given society would be given a certain number of stamps entitling him to, say, 1.3 children, or 0.8 children—which he could barter for other privileges (or vice versa).

Juniper, again, feels that what is required is "a device performing a contraceptive function that is constantly reliable, of micro-dimensions, both invisible and undetectable to the woman or man, that requires no servicing, that is difficult to tamper with, save with expert skill, and that lasts a woman's child-bearing lifetime, or a man's fertility period." Such concerns imply that children must begin getting contraceptive education at a very early age in order to prevent too many inadvertent conceptions; a significant proportion of today's births are the result of accidental teen-age pregnancies. Plans such as these always set off—and properly so—all our automatic alarm responses.

As soon as a state begins to require licensing for any activity, those authorized to issue the licenses also feel authorized—indeed, duty-bound—to inquire into the qualifications of (in this case) the potential parents, not to mention the quality of the potential offspring. Thus the family becomes politicized. After all, if a society is going to admit to its membership only a few new children in each generation, its leaders will want to be very selective. Under these conditions, children should be especially prized individuals, well cared for, nurtured, and educated under the benevolent surveillance, not merely of their own parents, but of the entire society. Yet the very concept of strict, compulsory birth limitation implies the total disqualification, and perhaps the enforced sterilization, of many people adjudged (by whom?) to be "unfit," or merely insufficiently perfect. It further implies compulsory genetic counseling, compulsory antenatal diagnosis, and, any time the outcome looks doubtful, compulsory abortion. (Most of us alive today might fail the admission requirements to such a society.)

As foreshadowed by Anthony Burgess's *The Wanting Seed,* in order to achieve population control homosexuality might be encouraged, heterosexual coupling discouraged, and "Mother" become a dirty word not only in jokes about psychoanalysts. The decision makers—the brave new society's equivalent of Huxley's Predestinators—may well decide that sexual intercourse is no longer the ideal civilized means for human propagation. They may opt for *in vitro* fertilization of selected donor eggs and sperm, perhaps pre-frozen, the cloning of cells taken from preselected individuals, and the use of other advanced procreative biotechnologies. The late Nobel geneticist Hermann Müller was a vocal advocate of "adoptive parenthood" rather than old-style genetic parenthood, where people self-ishly choose to perpetuate their own names and images rather than to have children with more suitable genetics. In an era when the genetic program for aging is under human control, the capacity should also be on hand for genetically programming most individuals to be infertile, if we so chose. In what form would the family survive? Would children be reared by the state or community rather than by individual parents? How would this affect the character of citizens that resulted? Which human qualities might be lost, and which gained? All these speculations—and they do not begin to exhaust even the obvious possibilities—reverberate with worrisome overtones.

To cryonicists and immortalists like Ettinger, Esfandiary, and Saul Kent (author of *Future Sex*), such worries are not taken too seriously. A major motif that runs through many of their arguments is that human nature, as well as the human social context, will have undergone such great changes that any extrapolations from present standards are simply meaningless. Indeed, when we consider how radically our standards have changed in the past decade or two *without* the application of any advanced biotechnology (unless one puts The Pill in that category) or any widespread immortalist hopes or beliefs—and, further, how rapidly the new standards (or lack of them) have been accepted—it would seem foolhardy to brush aside too summarily the case for much more drastic transformations ahead. Such science fiction seers as Arthur Clarke, Isaac Asimov, and Olaf Stapledon have imagined futures whose highly evolved, galactic-voyaging inhabitants are hardly recognizable as their former human selves.

To think seriously about the implications of an extended life span, however, one does not have to project one's scenarios into the scarcely imaginable future, or even to global concerns closer to us in time such as pollution and overpopulation. On an immediate personal, community, and national level, extended life would have a profound impact. We are hardly aware of how much of our thinking, our life patterns, and our social institutions depend on the assumed immutability of the human life span. One need only take a superficial look at some built-in assumptions of our economy to get a quick idea of the magnitude of the consequences.

Suppose only a modest number of vigorous years have been added to the average person's life. Think what might happen to Social Security programs, retirement benefits, insurance commitments. All such plans are predicated on making payments for a strictly limited number of years. Think of the Veterans Administration budget if war veterans did not die off but went on and on expecting a continuation of their compensatory payments for unlimited periods of time. Think of a city like New York, already reeling from the financial burden of paying lifetime retirement benefits to its still-young twenty-year retirees, still making payments to those same people, who may look and feel as young as ever long after one would have expected to attend their funerals. Each working generation would be supporting several generations of retired people simultaneously. Obviously adjustments and revisions would have to be made. The same would be true of all insurance contracts. If life expectancies go way up, should insurance premiums not come way down? Would long-lived, healthy people feel the need for insurance at all, except for special circumstances? Long-term loans, with interest piling on interest over the years, would of course require the setting of upper limits. All our economic programs might need extensive overhauling, if not complete redrafting.

In a society where old people not only lived longer but remained in such well-preserved condition as to be hardly distinguishable from the young in vigor and appearance, unfamiliar attitudes and relationships would evolve, new hopes and opportunities would arise, as well as new frustrations and resentments. Young people, even those who love and respect their elders, look to the day when those elders will step down from their positions, retire from active competition, die. They wait their turn, not always too patiently, for jobs, status, inheritance.

If a man or woman at sixty-five expected to remain vigorous and healthy for, say, another sixty-five or more years, current retirement policies would be mightily resisted and probably have to be changed. (It is possible this dilemma might be solved by "retiring" people into some other career; though there can be no assurance that openings would be more plentiful in other fields.) Healthy old people might be as unwilling to give up possessions as positions. The longer they lived, the less willing they would be. The power and wealth they could accumulate over a long lifetime would be formidable.

At present the old can give up their jobs and their status with a modicum of grace and good cheer because they know they cannot hope to do those jobs or take advantage of benefits for much longer anyway. They can leave fortunes to their heirs and to charitable institutions because they know that "you can't take it with you." They generally cherish the young—or at least the young to whom they are personally related, especially their own children. But how much of this feeling is based on the desire to see their names and images carried on in the next generation?

These feelings are bound to undergo some changes with increased longevity. If people begin more and more to think of themselves as their own heirs, how will it affect their attitudes toward their children —and vice versa? If people no longer needed to worry about the early decline of health and strength, would they continue to cherish and cultivate those who, they hope, will be their future caretakers? And if they can carry on their own names and images indefinitely, in person, what need for others to carry them vicariously? It may be, of course, that no matter how long life lasts, people will still worry about the end of it, will still want the assurance of closely related and caring people—though some futurists insist that all humankind should exercise the same kind of caring concern for all its members without the need for "blood" ties or genetic relationships.

It would be a puzzling experience indeed for young people to live in a world where old people did not age. At present, young people at least have the advantage of their youthful looks and energies. They can overwhelm their elders in almost any sport, in any contest of physical strength or endurance, and, usually though not invariably, in any competition for the sexual favors of attractive partners. If older people retained their own youthful exuberance, these compensatory advantages might all evaporate. And if the old had youth as well as wealth and power, displacing them might be almost beyond competitive hope. The young would increasingly resent and abhor the presence of these perpetually youthful monopolists—unless the latter could figure out a means of sharing their benefits without threatening their own welfare.

Juniper suggests that "an immortalist might not be allowed to amass wealth beyond a set figure or after a certain time. He might be required to hand back to a central property pool, or make over to a common fund, wealth he had accumulated beyond a given limit." I suppose this idea is simply an extension of the precedents established by income and inheritance taxes. It is even likely that a limit might be placed on life spans, or, at least, on the length of time a given individual would be permitted to spend on earth. In that event, death control would go hand in hand with birth control. As population pressures, among other pressures, mounted to a critical point, an upper limit of, say, 200 or 300 years might be set, after which the lucky winner might have a choice of going to live in orbit (or another planet or asteroid), if space were available out there, or else . . .

Would people be any readier to depart after two or three centuries of life than they now are after three score and ten years? Or would they hold life more dear than ever? We have no way of knowing, though here again there would probably be a spectrum of individual reactions. As we have seen, visionary types all the way from Pindar to Condorcet to Alan Harrington have assumed a new serenity in our attitudes if we were no longer condemned to a fixed life span. But Ernest Becker quotes Jacques Choron to the contrary: "postponement of death is not a solution to the problem of the fear of death . . . there still will remain the fear of dying prematurely." And Becker himself, in *The Denial of Death,* says: "The smallest virus or the stupidest accident would deprive a man not of ninety years but of 900—and would be then ten times more absurd. Condorcet's failure to understand psychodynamics was forgivable, but not Harrington's today. If something is ten times more absurd it is ten times more threatening. In other words, death would be 'hyper-fetishized' as a source of danger, and men in the utopia of longevity would be even less expansive and peaceful than they are today!"

For those reluctant to go, would there be an automatic death sentence? Would we be willing to reinstitute capital punishment after finally convincing ourselves that this kind of social vengeance is uncivilized, even for criminals? Might there be special circumstances for requesting extensions? Would a trial be necessary? Might there be a thriving black market in false birth records? Wouldn't it be hard to keep track of people who were highly mobile for a couple of centuries, and prove their correct ages? Could we in any case really bring ourselves to carry out the death penalty when the condemned individuals had done no wrong, were still in the productive prime of life, still very much wanted to live, and had the support of others who loved them and also wanted them to live? Perhaps there could be a lesser penalty—an interruption rather than a termination of life via an indefinite stretch of hibernation.*

For people ready to die, there would be no difficulty. They would simply commit suicide by some approved method on schedule, as envisioned in some of the science-fictional futures—Heinlein's, for example. In a world where the life span had been extended, we would in any case perhaps be obliged to change our rigid views toward the act of suicide. It would probably no longer be considered either an immoral or a criminal act. My assumption is that, if it becomes possible to medicate or manipulate our bodies to enable ourselves to live longer, no one will require us to take advantage of the opportunity. We will be allowed to age and die in peace, as of yore, if that is our personal choice.

Some strange relationships might develop between the short-lived and the long-lived. And there might be objections to permitting people to age and die in the old way on the grounds that they would thus be unproductive and, moreover, represent an unfair drain on society's medical and custodial resources. In such a society, would people turn away from "ugly old people" even more than they do now? Now, at least, we see in old people our future selves and should therefore look upon them with greater sympathy. Or is it perhaps precisely because we see in them our future selves that we turn away from them, not wanting to be reminded of our fate? Among the more melancholy people in all of history will be those old people who may be still around when gerontological help arrives but who are themselves too far gone to help; the last generation condemned to age irreversibly and die as heretofore. The most optimistic gerontologists hope, of course, that, once answers are arrived at, progress may be swift enough to help everyone who wants to be helped.

Even now, there is much debate in progress concerning a patient's right to die if he wishes rather than to accept heroic biotechnological measures to keep him alive from one day to the next to the next when there is no real hope that he can pull through. In

---

* I would guess that cryonic suspension will not, in the long run—even if it works—prove the best means of preserving people intact over time. Chemically induced hibernation—the method used naturally by the African lungfish which so fascinated heart surgeon Henry Swan—at room temperature might be safer, less expensive, more efficient, and less damaging, once the techniques have been perfected.

a few responsible quarters there is even some support for the idea that any person, ill or not, who simply decides he does not feel like living any longer, should—after all efforts to revive his interest in life, including religious and psychiatric counseling, have failed—be not only permitted to end his life, but be helped to make his exit in as tranquil and merciful a fashion as possible. This is the view, for instance, of German Nobel laureate Max Delbrück, one of the physicists who made such important contributions to molecular biology. In an interview for the American Medical Association publication *Prism,* Irving S. Bengelsdorf asked Delbrück, "Would you then say that we cannot avoid using science and technology to control the termination of life?"

"Yes," Delbrück replied. "Further, I would suggest that our society provide 'suicide education' as it now provides birth control information. . . . Society must have free access to information about forms of suicide that are not too repulsive.

"The present thrust of our society," he continued, "is to prolong life as long as possible. But there is no inherent biological or cultural necessity for such an attitude. The taking of one's life should be a matter of maturity as it was during the last hours of Socrates, as so wonderfully described by Plato."

He cites the case of the Nobel physicist Percy W. Bridgman, who, at the age of eighty, terminally ill with cancer, shot himself and left behind a note that read: "It isn't decent for society to make a man do this thing himself."

Delbrück went on to discuss how and when such education might be carried out. In high school or college? No, that is perhaps too soon. "I would suppose that suicide education should be given to people at an age when the person begins to realize that his stay on earth is finite. I don't think you can talk seriously to people about how to leave a party when they are just getting there and they think it's going to be a great party."

Whether or not we think life is going to be a "great party" does of course have a lot to do with our desire to stay or leave. Just accepting life as a tolerably good party is usually enough. The suicidal person has, as a rule, either come to look upon life's party as a dismal bore not to be tolerated or his own condition such as to render the party no longer enjoyable for himself—as in the case of Bridgman or, say, Hemingway, neither of whom found life boring. There is every reason to believe that life in an immortalist age* would be a very interesting party indeed; I'll come back to that in a moment. But note Delbrück's emphasis on realizing that one's stay on earth is finite. If death were postponable and life's quality remained high, would he still advocate suicide education? Delbrück clearly does not have much faith in the promise of gerontology. In an earlier portion of the same interview, Delbrück does flatly say, "We are mortal and will remain so. What we accomplish by medical research is merely to shift the statistics in the causes of death."

In the case of an artificially extended life span, individuals would probably have a much clearer right to opt out when they felt they had lived long enough. It might simply be a matter of deciding to go off the life-prolonging medications or techniques, in which case the remainder of life might follow its natural course. Or perhaps the genetic aging clock might be reset and the leavetaker could meanwhile keep himself going full swing until the day the clock stopped. If cessation of medication were to entail a long-drawn-out period— especially a long-drawn-out period of deterioration and debility—he might look for a quicker exit, and perhaps society would feel he was entitled to it. It may even be that, if aging had been programmed out of the genes, the "fail-safe mechanism" removed, growing old would be very difficult even if desired. In either case, the only way to die rapidly would be to commit suicide. Ideally, perhaps, people should be able to live as long as they want, even indefinitely, but go gracefully when they choose (as Bernard Williams suggested), with society's blessing. Thinking such thoughts is a difficult and distasteful pastime currently; but in an age when the planet became over-crowded and potential parents were waiting for vacancies so they could have children, perhaps we could face the willing deaths of people who had lived as long as they pleased much more easily than we now cope with the pain-filled departures of loved ones who would wish to stay with us longer—and whose added years might enrich the world and all that dwell therein.

If we were to permit the deliberate ending of the lives even of healthy people in full possession of their faculties, one wonders how

* I use the phrase "immortalist age" loosely as a convenient way of talking about the period that begins with the first true, significant, artificial extension of the human life span and continuing through successive and more radical gerontological successes, whenever they may occur.

we might begin to feel, on a planet of finite size with limited resources, about the retarded, the crippled, those who by some official designation were deemed defective or imperfect. Might we find ourselves thinking more and more in "eugenic" terms and want to put these unfortunates "out of their misery" and not permit them to be "burdens to society"? Many people have already demonstrated their attraction to this kind of thinking, and we would do well to be on guard against it. Preventing hypothetical people from being conceived and born is not the same as putting existing individuals to death, and we place our humanity in jeopardy when we contemplate such measures. There is no reason why we should ever do less than our best for every individual born into the world—unless, perhaps, his being here represents anguish beyond reasonable expectation of tolerance—and at least let him live out his natural span of years as pleasantly as possible.

Let us return, for a moment, to the kind of "party" life might be in the event that gerontology achieves its major goals. An immortalist society would surely pose new identity crises for its citizens. It would also require revised definitions of life and death, of youth and age. All human relationships would undergo change or at least reappraisal, including working arrangements, personal friendships, doctor-patient relationships, political associations, religious affiliations, sexual and romantic relationships, marriage and parenthood. We know that all change is stressful, and we can count on many more changes coming about through new biotechnological options—many of which were spelled out in my earlier book, *The Second Genesis.* We will possess a variety of interim biomedical strategies for delaying death, such as the successful transplantation of donor organs, the implantation of artificial parts, perhaps the growth of organs *in vitro* and their regeneration *in vivo,* and surely the control of immunological disorders, cancer, and the degenerative diseases—and ultimately for overcoming senescence and prolonging the life span. We are likely, too, to develop a large measure of control over our brains and minds, enlarging their capacities enormously—through, for instance, biofeedback, cybernetics, and brain-computer communications—and considerably ameliorating those aspects of "mental illness" contributed by faulty physiology and biochemistry. We will have at our command, as already indicated, an armamentarium of procreative biotechnologies, each with its accompanying risks and benefits: antenatal diagnosis and therapy, and the whole range of birth control techniques—control of both fertility and infertility, artificial insemination, artificial enovulation, frozen egg and sperm banks, ova and ovary transplantation, parthenogenesis, androgenesis, superovulation, *in vitro* fertilization and *in vitro* gestation, cloning, genetic engineering, gene transplants, and gene therapy. We may well be in control of all the basic mechanisms of all life's processes, and thus trustees of our own further evolution.

Are we ready to take on such awesome responsibilities? Can we really hope to maintain our human qualities in an immortalist world? Do we not need a constant infusion of "fresh blood" and young minds to help us cope with the challenge of changing circumstances? Would we not all become rigid, stultified, "set in our ways," desirous of preserving what makes us comfortable? Would we cease to be creative and thus be incapable of social evolution?

And what of our biological evolution? Could it proceed if death were indefinitely postponable and the turnover of generations (with fewer members in each) were to slow down? What of Denckla's failsafe mechanism? How could the species continue to evolve, or even to survive, in the face of environmental modifications if there were insufficient replacement of individuals to allow genetic mutations to take place, and to be passed on?

In this chapter I have sought merely to offer a quick, provocative, impressionistic first sketch of the nature and extent of the consequences implicit in indefinite prolongevity. Even a superficial look at such dilemmas, however, is enough to make many people hold their heads and holler: "Good heavens, haven't we got enough problems already? Let's not do it!"

Should we not?

Chapter XXI

NEVERTHELESS—YES, WE SHOULD!

By now you have undoubtedly surmised my own strong advocacy of gerontological research—not necessarily of the immortalist philosophy (about which I feel neutral), but of the quest for ways to add good years to the human life span. My advocacy is based on the belief that the thrust in this direction is (a) probably inevitable and (b) certainly desirable. I shall try, in this last brief chapter, to explain why I harbor these convictions despite my concern about the consequences we have just been discussing. I do share many of the qualms and misgivings of those less enthusiastic about pushing ahead with an anti-aging program. The "flavor of anxiety" is certainly not missing from my own musings about the future. But that should be true of anyone's musings about the future—even without any considerations of gerontology or immortalism. We are pressed upon from all sides by a multiplicity of gut-wrenching dilemmas, all demanding simultaneous solutions. For the relatively foreseeable future, small increases in the good years of individual lives will surely not add more than a few percentage points of aggravation to such overriding concerns as, say, worldwide pollution and overpopulation. These concerns are of such magnitude, and such immediacy, that they will have to be dealt with and, to some reasonable degree, solved long before the gerontologists have stirred their ingredients into the mix.

Moreover, it would be a mistake to assume that all the ingredients will necessarily be troublesome to society. Some may, indeed, provide substantial side benefits. One ingredient that longevity could well add to the mix—an ingredient which, though neither tangible nor measurable, might help energize us toward the more rapid resolution of our dilemmas—is motivation. We earlier mentioned, for instance, the pessimism some people feel about inducing us to care about what happens to posterity. We may, however, suddenly find it much easier to relate to the future if we ourselves were to *become* posterity.

If individual human beings have a good chance of finding themselves still personally on the scene to suffer the consequences of pollution, overpopulation, and bungled statesmanship, they will be more likely to devote some attention to avoiding those consequences, just as many individuals (though not all) might consider changing their diets, habits, or even life styles in order to add a few healthy years to their lives under present circumstances. It is an old truism that proprietors, or even long-term tenants, take much better care of their houses and apartments than transient occupants of the same premises. Even those whose minds are centered on industrial or personal profits might take a different view of pollutants shooting up from smokestacks, of effluents being discharged into rivers, of oceanic oilspills, of pesticide-poisoned wildlife, and assorted associated blights; and might even take independent initiative toward speeding ameliorative and prophylactic measures without needing to be goaded by militant environmentalists and conservationists. It would after all be their own supply of breathable air, of drinking water, of food, of resources, of all the appurtenances of health, comfort, and convenience that were being endangered. In such case, as Juniper again observes, "for the first time man will have the power to be himself, to make his own evaluation of life, and the effect may be to create between him and earth a new non-clinging, non-changing bond. This will be a relationship of equals, and the result may be that man may develop an entirely new sense of personal commitment to earth—a brother-earth philosophy of deep and abiding dimension." The extension of one's own being into the indefinite future, together with the possibility of identifying personally with posterity, might go a long way toward motivating us to a new impatience with delays and dawdling—the exact opposite of Heinlein's eternal procrastinators.

Any forecast of how human beings are likely to behave in an imagined set of future circumstances is, by its very nature, problematical. But I would guess that Stephen Leacock's man in the asbestos suit represents an unwarrantedly gloomy forecast of how long-lived individuals will behave. It seems doubtful to me that men and women will become so lackadaisical, even if allowed to indulge themselves without limit, as to lose their sense of adventure entirely. At any time, under any conditions, only a minority of the population is inclined to take unusual risks, but it is a consistent and substantial minority. Many young women and men of, say, twenty or twenty-five, quite willingly lay their lives—or at least their limbs—on the line, not only in the service of good humanitarian causes or even for selfish gains, but often for the sheer sport of it, for the intrinsic thrill of taking the risk. To people so young, the fifty or sixty years of leftover life they are risking must seem like long stretches of life indeed; if it were longer, they would probably still risk it. Older people, too, risk portions of their lives that may grow increasingly precious to them. I believe we will always be trying things just because the idea happened to occur to us, that we will always climb mountains just because They Are There.

My intuitive feelings about these matters, of course, can in no way be documented, or justified through *a priori* analysis, and could turn out to be wildly mistaken. We know that the malleability of human nature, while not infinite, renders all predications about it untrustworthy. (It provides hope, too, against the pessimism of those who insist that "You can't change human nature.") Nevertheless, we will be well advised to imagine what scenarios we can, to guess at the spectrum of human options implied, and to assign probability values—where we can—to the attitudes we deem most likely to prevail under various circumstances.

I am convinced that most of today's human values, our traditional sense of what is right and good versus what we feel to be wrong and evil, will still serve us well in most of the futuristic scenarios we can envision—those scenarios, at least, which do not imply a totalitarian social fabric. Such a conviction may of course say more about my own programming than about future realities. And the human values I speak of are in any case, at any given time, more honored than practiced. But we should certainly exercise restraint, as we learn increasingly to manipulate our minds and characters, to see that we do not program ourselves out of the qualities we most wish to keep.

Some future-watchers have emphasized the unbounded hedonistic opportunities ahead, the royal play. But a narcissistic preoccupation with the self cannot dominate the characters of those who populate the future; they will have to possess a good measure of altruistic concern for their fellow beings, and for their still generously endowed, though finite, planetary abode in the universe. It is only in the last instant of geologic time that we have discovered the finiteness of our planet; and the fact that we have not yet, in that instant, solved the dilemmas which the discovery has raised is hardly an adequate reason for pessimism.

We have lived through a period of bewildering change, and there is every evidence that change in the future will be constant and often radical. Change, as we know, is painful, or at least stressful—even change for the good, change which we all applaud. "The leader who denies the pain of change," says George Leonard, "is fooling his followers or, what is worse, himself." We will be constantly readjusting to these changes and helping others, who are perhaps less able to cope, do likewise. The well-functioning individual needs to be neither too selfish nor too selfless. He should have a healthy ego and a great appetite for joy, but also a compassionate sensitivity to the needs of others. Some of that joy should be generated by the very exhilaration of meeting the challenges of change—and of freedom.

The new era could bring us totally unprecedented freedoms. But freedom often turns out to be among the more unwelcome of human gifts. Our enemy is whoever gives us the means really to do what we want to do—which forces us to decide what we want to do. Despite our vocal celebrations of freedom, we tend to run from it. We prefer to have decisions made for us, to feel the security of a known order. I have elsewhere suggested a new definition of a healthy person: one who is exhilarated by the challenge of freedom. Such healthy people —and, with luck, that will include most of us—can find solutions to our problems, or devise ways to move us confidently into the future, with the sense of purpose that will provide a firm flow of stability against a backdrop of change—especially if they live long enough. (We should not overlook the probability that some of our seemingly insoluble problems may become obsolete or irrelevant as we enter new human situations possessed of new knowledge and capacities. As one homely example, if we succeed in harnessing new and plentiful energies, there would no longer be an "oil crisis.")

I said a moment ago that I consider it virtually inevitable that anti-aging research programs will proceed, and that they will succeed. We will almost surely pursue the necessary lines of research for all the usual scientific and medical reasons. We do not know nearly enough about either the organism we inhabit or the diseases and impairments that afflict it: cancer, heart disease, stroke, arthritis, dia-

betes, genetic defects, immunological disorders, "mental" illness, a
variety of still prevalent infectious diseases. It is therefore unlikely
that we will abandon promising avenues of biomedical research
while so many millions of our fellow creatures continue to suffer
from these ailments—one or more of which will, as likely as not,
strike us down personally, sooner or later. It is unthinkable that we
would settle for what we now know, and for our present treatments.
In the absence of better alternatives, we blast the afflicted with lethal
doses of radiation, pickle them in large quantities of poisonous drugs,
perform surgery that is complex, expensive, time-consuming, and
often mutilative. Many disease victims are increasingly dependent
for their lives on unwieldy machinery and heroic intensive care.
Sometimes—as in the case of some birth defects—the care can be
no more than custodial and may last a lifetime. Enormous effort is
often expended for a tiny gain in added life that is often of dubious
quality.

To declare a moratorium on all biomedical research (which no
one I know of is seriously proposing) would be to condemn us
permanently to a medical way of life that is intended only as an
interim holding action pending the discovery of causes, cures, and
preventive measures that will render obsolete these therapeutic
extravaganzas. To attain the longer-range goals will not only be infinitely less costly in cash but infinitely more rewarding by any human criterion. The victims, instead of costing so much, will be
producing, earning, spending. Instead of needing to be cared for,
they will be able to take care of, and provide for, others—and
certainly for themselves. Many of our social goals are muddied by a
conflict of values; what is good for society may be bad for the individual, and vice versa. But in this instance the desired outcome
would serve both individual happiness and the good of the species.

For many good reasons, then, we will doubtless pursue the kinds
of research we have been describing in this book. The bundle of
biological information that we need to understand life, to cure
genetic diseases and defects, to discover the cause and cure of cancer
and the secrets of immunology, to overcome the major degenerative
disorders, is the same bundle of information that will reveal the
mechanisms of the aging process. We might as well accelerate success
by deliberately seeking the gerontological answers. (It is my view,
incidentally, that biological controls will also provide us with

hitherto unknown methods of generating energy and recycling wastes, and of creating substantial new sources of food supply.)

Once the knowledge is at hand, there will of course be those who will want to use it to extend their lives and postpone their deaths. Many may protest that they would never make use of it under any circumstances. Some may feel strongly, in fact, that no one else should be permitted to employ it for prolongevity purposes either. But when it becomes clear that the end result will be not merely an ever-growing population of the old and enfeebled, but rather a group of elderly men and women like none who preceded them, living for many more years in the vigorous possession of their powers—I believe that more and more people will wish this outcome for themselves and for those they love. And the arguments for preventing others from taking advantage of this knowledge to this end will grow steadily thinner.

Consider how we spend our lives (those of us who are not handicapped either by chronic illness or poverty): In our early lives, our development is generally directed by others. They "educate" us. If we are lucky, they help us develop in directions that are in harmony with what seem to be our natural inclinations. They prepare us to become creative citizens, to make whatever contributions we may be capable of making to the world. Then, typically, when we have reached the stage where we are considered educated, mature, ready for adulthood, we marry and begin to sire, bear, and rear the next generation—whose education and development we then undertake as our major responsibility. We may, during these energetic years, fulfill ourselves in terms of a career, though, for most people, that career turns out to be only a job, because if we are to consider ourselves responsible citizens, our first concern is to earn a living, pay the rent, buy the baby a new pair of shoes. (All that has its own undeniable rewards, of course.) During these "best years of our lives," we may—the male and female alike—forego many pleasures, postpone many activities and ambitions. To what end? To raise our children to *their* adulthood so they can go and do likewise.

Finally, our responsibilities are taken care of. We have seen our children through college, say, and we are able to turn our attention to ourselves (if we have not, by then, forgotten what we wanted to do, what those marvelous contributions were that we secretly hoped we might achieve to justify the time we spent on earth), to indulge ourselves somewhat with minimal guilt, to start using some of those creative capacities which our education and experience have prepared us for. We have finally acquired a modicum of seasoning and of wisdom. And we realize that our health and vigor are not what they once were. We see the signs that the organism has begun to deteriorate irreversibly. Just when we could best make use of a generous stretch of time, we become acutely aware of how little time is left us—and that awareness colors everything we think and do. We begin to be haunted by the specter of a decline into relative helplessness, a fear confirmed by what we see on all sides when we look at the plight of the elderly; and we are saddened by the tragedy of lost human potential.

In Čapek's play, one of the characters finally feels a great surge of sympathy for what Emilia Marty has done and, far from condemning her, he advocates the same longevity for all:

VITEK (*Standing up and coming to the center of the group*): We'll make the Makropoulos secret public.

KOLONATY: Oh, no! Not that!

VITEK: We'll give it to everybody! We'll give it to the people. Everyone—everyone has the same right to life. We live for such a short time. How insignificant! God! How insignificant it is to be a human being.

KOLONATY: Rubbish!

VITEK: No, gentlemen, it does mean something! Just consider—the human soul, brains, work, love—everything. Good God, what can a man do in sixty years! What does he enjoy? What does he learn? He doesn't even enjoy the fruit of the tree he has planted; he doesn't learn all that his predecessors knew; he doesn't finish his work; he dies, and he hasn't lived. Ah, God, but we live so insignificantly!

KOLONATY: Well, Vitek—

VITEK: And he hasn't had time for gladness, and he hasn't had time to think, and he hasn't had time for anything except a desire for bread. He hasn't done anything, and he hasn't known anything. No, not even himself. Why have you lived? Has it been worth the trouble?

KOLONATY: Do you want to make me cry?

VITEK: We die like animals. What else is immortality of the soul but a protest against the shortness of life? A human being is something more than a turtle or a raven; a man needs more time to live. Sixty years—it's not right. It's weakness, it's ignorance, and it's animal-like.

HAUK-SENDORF: Oh, my, and I am already seventy-six!

VITEK: Let's give everyone a three-hundred-year life. It will be the biggest event since the creation of man; it will be the liberating and creating anew of man! God, what man will be able to do in three hundred years! To be a child and pupil for fifty years; fifty years to understand the world and its ways, and to see everything there is; and a hundred years to work in; and then a hundred years, when we have understood everything, to live in wisdom, to teach, and to give example. How valuable human life would be if it lasted for three hundred years! There would be no fear, no selfishness. Everything would be wise and dignified. (*Wringing his hands.*) Give people life! Give them full human life!

In like manner, Shaw's Dr. Conrad Barnabas, in *Back to Methuselah,* propagandizes for an extended life span. (Curiously, he too fixes on 300 years as the ideal figure.) In trying to urge his prolongevity program on a couple of eminent politicians, he says: "We're not blaming you: you hadnt lived long enough. No more had we. Cant you see that three-score-and-ten, though it may be long enough for a very crude sort of village life, isnt long enough for a complicated civilization like ours? Flinders Petrie has counted nine attempts at civilization made by people exactly like us; and every one of them failed just as ours is failing. They failed because the citizens and statesmen died of old age or over-eating before they had grown out of schoolboy games and savage sports and cigars and champagne."

In his preface to the long and seldom-performed play, Shaw himself had this to say: "Men do not live long enough; they are, for the purposes of high civilization, mere children when they die. . . . Life has lengthened considerably since I was born; and there is no reason why it should not lengthen ten times as much after my death.

"This possibility came to me when history and experience had convinced me that the social problems raised by millionfold national populations are far beyond the political capacity attainable in three score and ten years of life by slowgrowing mankind. On all hands as I write the cry is that our statesmen are too old, and that Leagues of Youth must be formed everywhere to save civilization from them. But despairing ancient pioneers tell me that the statesmen are not old enough for their jobs . . . we have no sages old enough and wise enough to make a synthesis of these reactions, and to develop the magnetic awe-inspiring force which must replace the policeman's baton as the instrument of authority."

Are we talking here about prolonged life only for leaders, or potential leaders, selected as a special elite? Or are we talking about a longer life for everyone? For everyone, of course. But this idea seems to offend some who at first are attracted to the idea of life extension. Here again, the two plays from which I have just been quoting bear some interesting parallels.

When Čapek's Vitek once again says, "We must prolong the life of all," Prus replies, "No, only the life of the strong. The life of the most talented. For the common herd this short life is good enough." When Vitek remonstrates, Prus brushes him aside:

> PRUS: Please, I do not want to argue. The ordinary, small, stupid one surely does not die. He is everlasting. Littleness multiplies without ceasing, like flies and mice. Only greatness dies. Only strength and talent die—and cannot be replaced. We ought to keep it in our own hands. We can prolong the life of the aristocracy.
>
> VITEK: Aristocracy! Do you hear that? Privilege on life!
>
> PRUS: Only the best are important in life. Only the chief, fertile and executive men. I am not mentioning women, but there are in this world about ten or twenty, perhaps a thousand, men who are irreplaceable. We can keep them. We can develop in them superhuman reason and supernatural power. We can breed ten, a hundred or a thousand supermen—masters and creators. So, I say, select those who have the right to unlimited life.

Similarly, when Shaw's Franklyn Barnabas (Conrad's brother) starts to explain: "When we get matured statesmen and citizens—" the politician Lubin stops short and exclaims, "Citizens! Oh! Are the citizens to live three hundred years as well as the statesmen?" Conrad says, "Of course," and Lubin replies, "I confess that had not occurred to me." (*"He sits down abruptly,"* the dramatist's stage instructions read, *"evidently very unfavourably affected by this new light."*) The other politician, Burge, finally says, after some calculation, "It's out of the question. We must keep the actual secret to ourselves."

Most fiction that deals with the longevity theme does go on the assumption that the life-prolonging or rejuvenation therapies and medications will be difficult and expensive, and accessible therefore only to the wealthy or privileged few. In *Bug Jack Barron,* by Norman Spinrad, rejuvenation depends on the transplantation of glands from a child—who is killed by the operation. There is only a black market for the glands, and only rich old men to buy them. Fred Mustard Stewart's *The Methuselah Enzyme* features a Swiss surgeon in an out-of-the-way sanatorium, and wealthy old people whose added years are robbed from younger people. In fact, there is no reason why whatever drugs and treatments flow out of gerontological research should not, as Comfort believes, be as universally available as any other drug or treatment, and could be considerably less expensive than many now in use.

The case that Vitek and Conrad Barnabas make for an extended life span is not a ridiculous one. For those individuals who enjoy life, aging and death are authentic tragedies. And these can be society's tragedies as well—for, as we have already discussed, just when women and men reach a point in life where their wisdom and experience equip them to begin giving their best to the world; just when they have completed their family duties and are free to pursue their creative inclinations—this is when their energies fail, and body and brain begin to degenerate.

But suppose their bodies remained strong and their intellects sharp?

Most of the varieties of biological control we have discussed connote the manipulation of ourselves from the outside, or at least with outside assistance. But, biotechnics aside, we should not overlook the many new opportunities that already exist for extended and life-enriching experiences from within ourselves. They lie in a heightened awareness of our own relatively untapped inner resources, as represented by the more worthwhile aspects of the still rather amorphous "human potential" and "new consciousness" movements, which go by various names. Many techniques have been employed to bring about the desired results: drugs, altered states of consciousness, physical and spiritual exercises, meditation, the Oriental martial arts, biofeedback, sensory deprivation, psychedelic environments—and the just plain straightforward opening up of people's awareness by pointing out unsuspected realities and potentials. Writing about these experiments in *Saturday Review,* Jean Houston (who, with her collaborator-husband Robert Masters, heads the Foundation for Mind Research) proposes a "psychenaut program,"* the aim of which would be "to put the first man on earth." The psychenaut program would be an "exploration of inner space." It would "map the mind and tap its unrealized capacities. It would acquaint the psychenauts with the phenomenal contents of their own beings—their mind-body systems [with more emphasis on the body than is customary in Western culture]—and teach them to employ and to enjoy the multiplicity of human qualities that seem almost unattainable on first encounter. Through intensive training, psychenauts would have new control over their creative energies, their health, their experience of time and space, heat and cold, pain and pleasure.

"This exploration of the farther reaches of human consciousness," Houston continues, "typifies a new kind of mind research, already well begun." She makes clear, too, that the psychenauts she is referring to will not be an elite handful of superpeople; they will rather be masses of ordinary women and men, but aware and awakened in an unprecedented manner. Thus future life could feasibly be not only as enjoyable as present life, but much more so.

As George Leonard agrees, in *The Transformation,* "Any decisive outward movement of human consciousness requires an equal and opposite movement to greater depths. In the long run, there can be no successful outer trip without an inner trip." One revelation of the inner trip: "We are strange and radiant creatures, flesh of the sun's flesh, most favored visible heirs of the primal consciousness."

The potential splendors of the upcoming era, even without "the immortality factor," have been delineated in shimmering terms by recent philosophers and sages all the way from Teilhard de Chardin to Sri Aurobindo. Leonard has called this period just ahead The Transformation; I have called it Genesis II; Boulding—in *The Meaning of the Twentieth Century*—labeled it "post-civilization" (to be inhabited, perhaps, by Sir Julian Huxley's "trans-humans"); Jonas Salk has given it a name that may have the best chance of sticking—Epoch B (in contrast with Epoch A, denoting all of human history until now)—and has, in *The Survival of the Wisest,* supplied us with some guidance as to how to make it come about.

* In 1969, in his presidential address to the American Psychopathological Association, Joel Elkes of Johns Hopkins University, a pioneer psychopharmacologist, proposed a quite similar "intronaut program," stressing the need for "inner space laboratories" soundly grounded in psychobiological research.

The promise of space—orbital space, the moon, the planets, and beyond—has provided a heady set of goals for many: among them, Wernher von Braun and Neil Armstrong, Krafft Ehricke and Gerard O'Neil, Earl and Barbara Hubbard.

Even without dreaming of extraterrestrial travel or colonization, without seeking the delight to be provided by the new expansions of consciousness, many people would quite happily settle for more of the same, especially if endowed with reasonably good health and adequate means. To have time to travel everywhere, and go back again and again to favorite places. To go on learning— new skills, new sports, new languages, new musical instruments. To undertake a variety of careers and a diversity of relationships; for some, perhaps, a diversity of marriages. To read everything you want to read. To listen to all the music. To look at all the pictures, and even paint a few. To savor and re-savor experience and arrive, not at boredom but at new levels of appreciation. To be around long enough to use your talents to make some contribution to the world.

But what of the consequences, expressed earlier, of an insufficiency of "fresh blood"—and therefore of fresh thinking—in terms of discouraging creativity? The immortalist hope is that people who live longer will become wiser, that their continued vigor will keep them thinking freshly and creatively, that the mature individual—no longer prey to energy-draining anxiety over his failing powers—will save his anxiety for the future of his species (especially since he will be the personal sharer of that future). The definition of that species, as Leonard suggests, might be expanded to include all life on earth—at least, until life is discovered elsewhere. Moreover, children would continue to be born, though in diminished numbers; and it is assumed that, rather than being looked upon as new-arriving upstarts and competitors, they would be especially nourished, cherished, and encouraged to develop, in mind and body, their maximum human potential in the most congenial possible educational milieu. Thus, fresh thinking *would* continue to arrive, the quantity lessened but the quality undoubtedly improved. "Up to now," writes Leonard, "death has served as a primary mechanism of evolution, from the lower organisms up through humankind in society. . . . When the time comes—as it may well be coming—that individual human organisms can truly change and go on changing in ways that now seem hardly possible, when they can create and go on creating ever-changing cultures, then death will have lost its function where human evolution is concerned." Leonard, whose attention has not been particularly centered on aging or immortality, goes on to add: "Realizing and questioning its [death's] utility, we should not be caught by surprise when we find that aging can be greatly slowed or even stopped."

Dean Juniper, too, questions whether "the youth-versus-age combination is vital in keeping up a flow of new ideas. Flexibility of contact between creative individuals and creative groups does seem to be essential. But given the fact that all creative persons would retain their physical and intellectual powers indefinitely it would seem immaterial how continuous cross-fertilization came about, provided it came about. Thus an immortalist society which deliberately set out being creative might end up more creative by design than it might ever have been by natural accident."

As for biological evolution, we know that most mutations are deleterious and only a minority contribute to positive evolution; and employing nature's clumsy, trial-and-error method, individuals sicken, suffer, and die in large numbers in order that the species may adapt and survive through the vicissitudes of environmental change. In the age of longevity, with genetic engineering at our service, perhaps we could create our own mutations with greater efficiency and incalculably less human misery (though of course we could cause incalculably more if we use our knowledge foolishly). Hence we would have no further need of the built-in fail-safe mechanisms we have called aging and death.

There is no telling what a man or woman might become or achieve in a significant number of extra years. It is not just that an individual who lived for a very long time could learn more facts and more skills, but that he could consolidate and synthesize his learning in altogether new ways. He could go back over and over his varied and ever-expanding knowledge and continue to make new connections. He could resynthesize, in collaboration with similar long-livers, whole new systems of thought, bringing together mathematics, physics, astronomy, cosmology, geology, meteorology, chemistry, paleontology, archeology, biology, psychology, medicine, anthropology, sociology, economics, history, politics, art, literature, drama, poetry, music, theology, law, philosophy—the entire catalog of human disciplines and indisciplines, plus others yet to be created; the grand union of simultaneous-multitudinous connectedness that Hesse could only hint at in the intricate "glass bead game" of *Magister Ludi*.

One of the highest talents of such an individual might be creative mythologizing. We are in constant need of myths to live by as Joseph Campbell, among others, has tirelessly emphasized. And by "myth" I do not mean a fanciful story or framework which we must accept purely on faith, with no evidence to support it; but rather a *likely* myth which works for us because we believe in it. And we believe in it because it fits the knowledge we possess at any given time—or at least does not contradict it in a way that grossly affronts our intelligence. Much of this knowledge, though certainly not all of it, may be acquired through science. Because such knowledge must remain incomplete, at least for any time ahead that we can foresee, it can seldom if ever be absolute in nature; it must remain to some extent tentative, subject to revision on the arrival of new insights or more reliable data. But our knowledge could still have high probability value as pragmatic truth to live by, within a creatively structured mythological context that could answer our deeply felt spiritual longings and permit us to maintain hope, self-esteem, and a sense of purpose. The kind of long-lived individual I have just been hypothesizing, armed with an understanding of probabilistic reasoning as well as a due respect for the irrational in our natures, might be ideally equipped to create such vital myths for us. It is not unreasonable to hope that such human seers (by current standards) might even provide us with viable political solutions to which our present limitations blind us.

There could arise a new breed of human being who, merely by virtue of his longevity, through the acquisition of a steadily maturing wisdom and a steadily expanding awareness, could finally become exactly the kind of gifted individual we need to help take our species into a challenging and expanded future—a being to whom we might entrust the decisions that go with controlling the mechanisms of life, a being worthy to be the trustee of our further evolution to a destiny of our own choosing.

What has always prevented any serious, widespread consideration of such questions is the long-standing and continuing lack of credibility that such questions would ever truly *become* serious. As Shaw's Lubin finally says to Franklyn Barnabas: "I grant you that if we could live three hundred years we should all be, perhaps wiser, certainly older. You will grant me in return, I hope, that if the sky fell we should all catch larks."

It is difficult to consider seriously a proposal which is impossible of attainment. And everybody has always "known"—except for a few cranks and crackpots—that extending the human life span is and always will be a pipedream. That is why I have devoted the major space in this book to spelling out the research and theories that suddenly transform the pipedream into at least a feasible fantasy, and perhaps a reality we can plan for. Unlike Shaw's Barnabas, who was relying on the sheer power of wishful thinking to bring about his extended life span, we will soon have in our hands the biological tools to bring about, in a practical manner, the long-sought elixir of life, in one form or another. Old age will be a disease you can go see your doctor about, if, indeed, prophylactic measures do not virtually eradicate it.

Our species is at a critical transition point in its history on this planet. To fear the consequences of further knowledge—and thus decide to halt further research—would be the surest road to a non-solution of our problems, and thus to disaster. We do not begin to know all that we need to know. Why not take up, with some anticipatory exhilaration, the challenge of pursuing whatever path may bring us to our full humanhood?

The fact that we must work with incomplete knowledge should not deter us from moving ahead with high spirits—always tempered, to be sure, by a reasonable caution. To the basic question of epistemology, we must answer that the knowledge we possess or can realistically hope to acquire has its limitations. But we do not begin to know what those limitations are, and we may properly assume that in the next phase of our evolution, and the next, the scope of our understanding will continue to be enlarged. With this enlargement there may emerge startlingly different views of reality, of the way we perceive the universe and ourselves.

To the basic question of teleology, we must admit that we do not know with any certainty if there is purpose in the universe (unless we accept it as given via any of our religions); or, if so, what that purpose is; or where we fit into it either as a species or as individuals. Nevertheless, I do not agree with those philosophers who adduce impeccable arguments to prove that there definitely is *not* any purpose in this random, entropic universe, nor any meaning to human life beyond an existential imperative to survive without illusions.* They are, at the least, arriving at premature conclusions based on the skimpiest of data. (I am thinking, for instance, of Jacques Monod's beautifully written and elegantly reasoned *Chance and Necessity*.) The teleological question must remain open. Meanwhile, it is not fatuous to believe that there is a purposeful thrust to what is happening, even though we are not (at least not yet) equipped to discern it. I like to think that one of life's purposes is to divine life's purpose.

I have talked somewhat glibly about controlling our own destiny and moving on to the next stage of evolution, to L. L. Whyte's "next development in man." But I would certainly prefer to see us postpone any hasty moves to that next evolutionary phase, which we can at best only dimly perceive, until we have firmly consolidated our present phase. We must learn to be truly human first. To do that, however, will still require that we transcend our present selves in ways that will demand all the courage, compassion, imagination, good sense, and good cheer that we can muster. And the mustering of those resources would, I think, be considerably enhanced by the addition of good years to good lives.

---

* It should be noted that I do not equate "illusion" with "myth" as I defined it earlier. Even if an existential view were warranted, I do not think it would inevitably lead us to either total absurdity or total despair—but that is another whole book.

Bibliography

Abu-Erreish, Ghaleb, and Sanadi, D. Rao. "Mitochondrial Structure and Function in Aging." Prepublication abstract.
————. Neely, James R., et al. "Studies in Fatty Acid Oxidation by Isolated Perfused Working Hearts of Aged Rats." Prepublication abstract.
Adelman, Richard C. "Enzyme Adaptation in Aging." Presented at American Association for the Advancement of Science, San Francisco, 1974.
————. "Impaired Hormonal Regulation of Enzyme Activity during Aging." Prepublication manuscript for *Federation Proceedings,* 1974.
————, and Britton, Gary W. "The Impaired Capability for Biochemical Adaptation During Aging." *BioScience,* Oct. 1975.
Adler, William H. "Aging and Immune Function." *BioScience,* Oct. 1975.
Allfrey, Vincent G., and Mirsky, Alfred E. "How Cells Make Molecules." *Scientific American,* Sept. 1961.
Altman, Lawrence K. "Gain Reported in Halting Aging in Cells." *New York Times,* Sept. 20, 1974.
————. "Protein Found in Elderly Studied for Link to Aging." *New York Times,* Oct. 22, 1973.
Andres, Reubin. Personal interview.
————. "Defining and Evaluating the Myriad Influences on Human Aging." *Geriatrics,* March 1975.
Andron, Leo A., II, and Strehler, Bernard L. "Recent Evidence on tRNA and tRNA Acylase-Mediated Cellular Control Mechanisms: A Review." *Mechanisms of Ageing and Development,* Vol. 2, 1973.
Ascheim, P. "Résultats fournis par la greffe heterochrone des ovaires dans l'étude de la régulation hypothalamo-hypophyso-ovarienne de la ratte senile." *Gerontologia,* Vol. 10, 1964/1965.

Asimov, Isaac. "The Coming Age of Age." *Prism*, Jan. 1975.
————. "Why We Must Grow Old." *Science Digest*, Dec. 1970.
Atlan, Henri, Miquel, Jaime, and Binnard, Rosemarie. "Differences Between Radiation-Induced Life Shortening and Natural Aging in *Drosophila Melanogaster*." *Journal of Gerontology*, Jan. 1969.
Austin, James H. Personal communications.
Bailey, A. J., Robins, S. P., and Balian, G. "Biological Significance of the Intermolecular Crosslinks of Collagen." *Nature*, Sept. 13, 1974.
Balazs, A. "Organismal Differentiation, Ageing and Rejuvenation." *Experimental Gerontology*, Oct. 1970.
Barrows, Charles H., Jr. "The Challenge—Mechanisms of Biological Aging." *The Gerontologist*, Spring 1971.
————. "Ecology of Aging and of the Aging Process—Biological Parameters." *The Gerontologist*, Summer 1968.
Bean, William B. Personal conversations.
————. "Nail Growth: A Twenty-Year Study," *Archives of Internal Medicine*, April 1963.
Becker, Ernest. *The Denial of Death*. New York: The Free Press (Macmillan), 1973.
Bender, A. D., Kormendy, C. G., and Powell, R. "Pharmacological Control of Aging." *Experimental Gerontology*, Vol. 5, 1970.
Benet, Sula. *How to Live to Be 100: The Life-Style of the People of the Caucasus*. New York: Dial Press, 1976.
Benson, Andrew A. Personal communication.
Beregi, Edit. "Morphology of Antibody-Forming Cells in Young and Aged Experimental Animals." *Mechanisms of Ageing and Development*, Vol. I, 1972.
Berg, Paul, Baltimore, David, et al. "Asilomar Conference on Recombinant DNA Molecules." *Science*, June 6, 1975, and *Nature*, June 5, 1975.
Bernstein, Seldon. Personal conversation.
Beverley, E. Virginia. "Exploring the Many-Faceted Mysteries of Aging." *Geriatrics*, March 1975.
Bierman, Edwin L. "Aging, Metabolism and Atherosclerosis." *Guidelines to Metabolic Therapy*, Winter 1974.
Bilder, Glenda E., and Denckla, W. Donner. "Restoration of Juvenile Competence in Immune and RE Systems After Hypophysectomy of Adult Rats." Prepublication manuscript.
Birren, James E., ed. *The Relations of Development and Aging*. Springfield, Ill.: Charles C Thomas, 1964.
————. *Handbook of Aging and the Individual, Psychological and Biological Aspects*. Chicago: University of Chicago Press, 1959.
————. "Research on Aging: A Frontier of Science and Social Gain."

Presented to Senate Subcommittee on Government Research, Oct. 24, 1966.

Bjorksten, Johan. Personal communications.

——. "Crosslinkage as a Lead in Aging Research." Paper presented at Symposium on Theoretical Aspects of Aging, University of Miami, Feb. 6–8, 1974.

——. "The Crosslinkage Theory of Aging." *Finska Kemists. Medd.*, Vol. 80, No. 2, 1971.

——. "Approaches and Prospects for the Control of Age-Dependent Deterioration." *Annals of the New York Academy of Sciences,* June 7, 1971.

——. "The Crosslinkage Theory of Aging." *Journal of the American Geriatrics Society,* April 1968.

——. "Enzymes and Aging," in *Enzymes in Mental Health.* Edited by Gustav J. Martin and Bruno Kisch. Philadelphia: J. B. Lippincott, 1966.

——. *Thirteen-Year Report* (*1952–1965*) *of the Studies on Aging.* Bjorksten Research Foundation.

——. "Why Grow Old?" *Chemistry,* June 1964.

——. "Chemical Causes of the Aging Process." *Proceedings of the Scientific Section of The Toilet Goods Association,* May 1964.

——. "Aging, Primary Mechanism." *Gerontologia,* Vol. 8, 1963.

——. "Aging: Present Status of Our Chemical Knowledge." *Journal of the American Geriatrics Society,* Feb. 1962.

——. "A Common Molecular Basis for the Aging Syndrome." *Journal of the American Geriatrics Society,* Oct. 1958.

Bondareff, William, and Narotzky, Robert. "Age Changes in the Neuronal Microenvironment." *Science,* June 9, 1972.

Bonner, James. Personal communications.

——. *The Molecular Biology of Development.* New York and Oxford: Oxford University Press, 1965.

——. "Beyond Man's Genetic Lottery." Prepublication manuscript.

Borek, Ernest. *The Sculpture of Life.* New York: Columbia University Press, 1973.

——. "tRNA and Ageing." *Nature,* Sept. 20, 1974.

Bortz, Edward L. *Creative Aging.* New York: Macmillan, 1963.

——, and Walter M., II. "Major Issues of Aging." *GP,* July 1959.

Boulding, Kenneth. "Is Science Reaching the Point of a Diminishing Return?" *International Herald Tribune,* Sept. 7, 1970.

Boyer, Samuel H., Siggers, David C., and Krueger, Leslie J. "Caveat to Protein Replacement Therapy for Genetic Disease: Immunological Implications of Accurate Molecular Diagnosis." *The Lancet,* Sept. 22, 1973.

Brady, Roscoe O., Pentchev, Peter G., et al. "Replacement Therapy for

Inherited Enzyme Deficiency." *The New England Journal of Medicine,* Nov. 7, 1974.

Brekhman, I. I. "Ancient Ginseng and Pharmacology of the Future." Prepublication manuscript.

————, and Dardymov, I. V. "Pharmacological Investigation of Glycosides from Ginseng and Eleutherococcus." *Lloydia,* March 1969.

Brody, Harold. Personal communication.

————. "A Study of Aging in the Human Cerebral Cortex." *Journal of Comparative Neurology,* Vol. 102, 1955.

Brownlee, G. G. "Genetic Engineering with Viruses." *Nature,* Oct. 11, 1974.

Bucher, N. L. R., Scott, J. F., and Aub, J. C. "Regeneration of Liver in Parabiotic Rats." *Cancer Research,* Vol. 10, 1950.

Bullough, W. S. "Ageing of Mammals." *Nature,* Vol. 229, 1971.

Bunzel, Joseph H. "Recognition, Relevance and Deactivation of Gerontophobia: Theoretical Essay." *Journal of the American Geriatrics Society,* Vol. 21, No. 2, 1973.

Burnet, Sir F. Macfarlane. *Intrinsic Mutagenesis: A Genetic Approach to Aging.* New York: John Wiley & Sons, 1974.

————. *Genes, Dreams and Realities.* London: Pelican Books, 1973.

————. "A Genetic Interpretation of Ageing." *The Lancet,* Sept. 1, 1973.

Butler, Robert N. *Why Survive?—Being Old in America.* New York: Harper & Row, 1975.

————, ed. "Symposium on Mental Health and Aging: Life Cycle Perspectives." A special issue of *Geriatrics,* Nov. 1974.

————. "Age: The Life Review." *Psychology Today,* Dec. 1971.

Calloway, Nathaniel O. "Nutrition in Aging." Paper presented to American Association for the Advancement of Science, San Francisco, 1974.

Čapek, Karel. *The Makropoulos Secret.* Boston: International Pocket Library, 1925.

Caras, Roger. *Sockeye: The Life of a Pacific Salmon.* New York: Dial Press, 1975.

Carrel, Alexis. "On the Permanent Life of Tissues Outside of the Organism." *Journal of Experimental Medicine,* Vol. 15, 1912.

Casler, Lawrence. Personal communication.

————. "Psychosomatic Aspects of Death: An Experiment with Suggestive Therapy." Presented at American Psychological Association, Washington, 1967.

Chebotarev, D. F. Personal communication.

————. "Biological Active Agents ('Geriatrics') in Prevention and Treatment of Premature Aging," in *The Main Problems of Soviet Gerontology.* Kiev, 1972.

————, Ed. *The Main Problems of Soviet Gerontology.* Kiev, 1972.

————, Ed. "Longevous People (Physio-Clinical and Socio-Hygienic Research)." *Journal of the International Association on the Artificial Prolongation of the Human Specific Lifespan*, Vol. 1, No. 1, 1973.

Chen, Jenn C., Warshaw, Joseph B., and Sanadi, D. Rao. "Regulation of Mitochondrial Respiration in Senescence." *Journal of Cellular Physiology*, Aug. 1972.

Cherry, Rona and Cherry, Laurence. "Slowing the Clock of Age," *New York Times Magazine*, May 12, 1974.

Chown, Sheila M., Ed. *Human Ageing* (Selected Readings). London: Penguin Books, 1972.

Claiborne, Robert. *God or Beast: Evolution and Human Nature.* New York: W. W. Norton, 1974.

Clarke, Arthur C. *Profiles of the Future: An Inquiry into the Limits of the Possible.* New York: Harper & Row, 1962.

Clemens, J. A. and Meites, J. "Neuroendocrine Status of Old Constant-Estrous Rats." *Neuroendocrinology*, Vol. 7, 1971.

Cohen, Charles M., Weissmann, Gerald, et al. "Introduction of Purified Hexosaminidase A into Tay-Sachs Leukocytes by Means of Immuno-globulin-Coated Liposomes." Prepublication manuscript.

Colon, E. J. "The Elderly Brain: A Quantitative Analysis in the Cerebral Cortex of Two Cases." *Psychiatria, Neurologia, Neurochirurgia*, Vol. 75, 1972.

Comfort, Alex. Personal conversations and communications.

————. *The Nature of Human Nature.* New York: Harper & Row, 1966.

————. *Ageing: The Biology of Senescence.* New York: Holt, Rinehart & Winston, revised 1964.

————. "The Position of Aging Studies." *Mechanisms of Ageing and Development*, Vol. 3, 1974.

————. "So You Want to Live Longer." *Observer Magazine*, Sept. 23, 1973.

————. "Neuromythology?" *Nature*, Jan. 22, 1971.

————. "To Be Continued." *Playboy*,

————. "The Prospects for Age Control." Prepublication manuscript.

————. "The Prospects for Living Even Longer." Interview in *Time*, Aug. 3, 1970.

————. "The Biological Basis for Increasing Longevity." *Medical Opinion & Review*, April 1970.

————. "Test-Battery to Measure Ageing-Rate in Man." *The Lancet*, Dec. 27, 1969.

————. "The Prevention of Ageing in Cells." *The Lancet*, Dec. 17, 1966.

————. "Longevity of Man and His Tissues," in *Man and His Future*. Boston: Little Brown, 1963.

Costanzi, John J., and Goldstein, Allan L. "Immunotherapy: New Hope for the Cancer Patient." *Family Physician*, Vol. 8, 1973.

Cowdry, E. V. *Aging Better,* Springfield, Ill.: Charles C Thomas, 1972.

Cousins, Norman. *The Celebration of Life.* New York: Harper & Row, 1974.

Crick, F. H. C. "The Genetic Code: III." *Scientific American,* Oct. 1966.

———. "The Genetic Code." *Scientific American,* Oct. 1962.

———. "The Structure of Hereditary Material." *Scientific American,* Oct. 1954.

Curtin, Sharon R. *Nobody Ever Died of Old Age.* Boston: Little, Brown & Co., 1972.

Curtis, Howard J. *Biological Mechanisms of Aging.* Springfield, Ill.: Charles C Thomas, 1966.

Danes, B. Shannon. "Progeria: a Cell Culture Study on Aging." *Journal of Clinical Investigation,* Vol. 50, 1971.

Danielli, James F. Personal communications.

——— and Muggleton, Audrey. "Some Alternative States of Amoeba, with Special Reference to Life Span." *Gerontologia,* Vol. 3, 1959.

Davies, David. "A Shangri-la in Ecuador." *New Scientist,* Feb. 1, 1973.

Dawkins, Richard. "Selective Neurone Death as a Possible Memory Mechanism." *Nature,* Jan. 8, 1971.

de Beauvoir, Simone. *The Coming of Age.* New York: G. P. Putnam's Sons, 1972.

DeBusk, Franklin L. "The Hutchinson-Gilford Progeria Syndrome." *Journal of Pediatrics,* April 1972.

deDuve, Christian. "Lysosomes and Aging." Paper presented to American Association for the Advancement of Science, San Francisco, 1974.

Delbrück, Max. "Education for Suicide." Interview in *Prism,* Nov. 1974.

Denckla, W. Donner. Personal interviews and communications.

———. *The Physician and Man's Fate,* printed brochure.

———. "A Time to Die." *Life Sciences,* Vol. 16, 1974.

———. "Role of the Pituitary and Thyroid Glands in the Decline of Minimal O_2 Consumption with Age." *Journal of Clinical Investigation,* Feb. 1974.

———. "Ions, Energy and Aging." Prepublication manuscript.

deRopp, Robert S. *The New Prometheans.* New York: Dell Publishing Co., 1972.

———. *Man Against Aging.* New York: St. Martin's Press, 1960.

Dewey, Patrick R. Personal communication.

———. Editorials in *The Outlook.*

Dilman, V. M. "Age-Associated Elevation of Hypothalamic Threshold to Feedback Control, and Its Role in Development, Ageing, and Disease." *The Lancet,* June 12, 1971.

Dobzhansky, Theodosius. *The Biology of Ultimate Concern.* New York: World Publishing, 1969.

——. *Mankind Evolving: The Evolution of the Human Species.* New Haven, Conn.: Yale University Press, 1962.

Donovan, Jim. "Thymosin: Wonder Drug of the Seventies?" *University Medical,* Jan.–Feb. 1975.

Doty, Paul. "Proteins." *Scientific American,* Sept. 1957.

Doy, C. H., Gresshoff, P. M., and Rolfe, B. G. "Biological and Molecular Evidence for the Transgenosis of Genes from Bacteria to Plant Cells." *Proceedings of the National Academy of Science,* March 1973.

Dubos, René. Personal conversations.

——. *Beast or Angel? Choices That Make Us Human.* New York: Charles Scribner's, 1974.

——. *A God Within.* New York: Charles Scribner's, 1972.

——. *So Human an Animal.* New York: Charles Scribner's, 1968.

——. *Man Adapting.* New Haven, Conn.: Yale University Press, 1965.

Dykhuizen, Daniel. "Evolution of Cell Senescence, Atherosclerosis and Benign Tumors." *Nature,* Oct. 18, 1974.

Edson, Lee. "A Secret Weapon Called Immunology." *The New York Times Magazine,* Feb. 17, 1974.

——. "Genes: Altering the Cell—The Vistas Are Breathtaking." *New York Times,* Oct. 31, 1971.

Elgin, Sarah C. R. and Weintraub, Harold. "Chromosomal Proteins and Chromatin Structure." *Annual Reviews of Biochemistry,* 1975.

Epstein, J., Williams, Jerry R., and Little, John B. "Deficient DNA Repair in Human Progeroid Cells." *Proceedings of the National Academy of Sciences,* April 1973.

Erbe, Richard W. "Therapy in Genetic Disease." *The New England Journal of Medicine,* Nov. 7, 1974.

Erlanger, M., and Gershon, D. "Studies on Aging in Nematodes—II. Studies of the Activities of Several Enzymes as a Function of Age." *Experimental Gerontology,* March 1970.

Esfandiary, E. M. *Up-Wingers: A Futurist Manifesto.* New York: John Day, 1973.

——. *Optimism One.*

Ettinger, Robert C. W. Personal conversations and communications.

——. *Man Into Superman.* New York: St. Martin's Press, 1972.

——. *The Prospect of Immortality.* New York: Doubleday & Co., 1964.

——. "Cryonics and the Purpose of Life." *Christian Century,* Oct. 4, 1967.

Fabris, N., Pierpaoli, W., and Sorkin, E. "Lymphocytes, Hormones and Ageing." *Nature,* Dec. 29, 1972.

Feinberg, Gerald. *The Prometheus Project.* New York: Doubleday, 1968.

———. "Can We and Should We Do Anything to Prolong Youth?" Presented at Donnell Library Center, New York, Jan. 11, 1971.

Finch, Caleb. Personal interviews and communications.

———. "Neuroendocrinology of Aging: A View of an Emerging Area." *BioScience*, Oct. 1975.

———. "Hormones and Mammalian Ageing: A Synopsis." Prepared for Conference on Nutrition and Aging Processes, Seattle, 1973.

———. "The Regulation of Physiological Changes During Aging: A Hypothesis." Prepublication manuscript.

———. "Comparative Biology of Senescence: Evolutionary and Developmental Considerations." Prepublication manuscript.

Fishbein, Morris. "Psychogeriatrics in an Aging World." *Medical World News* (Editorial), Aug. 10, 1973.

Fletcher, Joseph. *The Ethics of Genetic Control*. Garden City, N.Y.: Doubleday Anchor Press, 1974.

Fletcher, M. J., and Sanadi, D. R. "Turnover of Rat Liver Mitochondria." *Biochimica et Biophysica Acta*, Vol. 51, 1961.

Frank, Benjamin S. Personal interviews and communications.

———. *Nucleic Acid Therapy in Aging and Degenerative Disease*. New York: Psychological Library Publishers, 1968.

———. "A Molecular Basis of Aging." Prepublication manuscript.

———. "Nucleic Acids, Aging and Oxygen." Prepublication manuscript.

Franks, L. M. "Cellular Aspects of Ageing." *Experimental Gerontology*, Oct. 1970.

Fridovich, Irwin. "Superoxide Dismutases." *Annual Reviews of Biochemistry*, 1975.

Friedman, D., Keiser, V., and Globerson, A. "Reactivation of Immunocompetence in Spleen Cells of Aged Mice." *Nature*, Oct. 11, 1974.

Friedman, Thomas B., Yarkin, Rhoda J., and Merril, Carl R. "Galactose and Glucose Metabolism in Galactokinase Deficient, Galactose–1–P–Uridyl Transferase Deficient and Normal Human Fibroblasts." *Journal of Cellular Physiology*, June 1975.

Froelich, Warren. "Aging Can Be Halted or Reversed 'In Our Generation,' Doctor Says." *Philadelphia Bulletin*, March 2, 1974.

Frolkis, V. V. "Functions of Cells and Biosynthesis of Protein in Aging." *Gerontologia*, Vol. 19, 1973.

———. "Acetylcholine Metabolism and Cholinergic Regulation of Functions in Aging." *Gerontologia*, Vol. 19, 1973.

———. "Regulation and Adaptation Processes in Aging." *The Main Problems of Soviet Gerontology*, Kiev, 1972.

———. "The Autonomic Nervous System in the Aging Organism." *Triangle*, The Sandoz Journal of Medical Science, Vol. 8, 1968.

———, Bezrukov, V. V., et al. "The Hypothalamus in Aging." *Experimental Gerontology*, Vol. 7, 1972.

————. "Catecholamines in the Metabolism and Functions Regulation in Aging." *Gerontologia*, Vol. 16, 1970.

Furukawa, Toshiyuki, Michitoshi, Inoue, et al. "Assessment of Biological Age by Multiple Regression Analysis." *Journal of Gerontology*, Vol. 30, No. 4, 1975.

Galton, Lawrence. *Don't Give Up on an Aging Parent.* New York: Crown Publishers, 1975.

Gardner, E. "Decrease in Human Neurones with Age." *Anatomical Record*, Vol. 77, 1940.

Garey, Walter (Project Manager). *R/V Alpha Helix Bering Sea Expedition, Feb.–Oct. 1968* and *Alpha Helix Research Program, 1972–1974.* Reports of the Scripps Institution of Oceanography, University of California at San Diego.

Geier, Mark R. Personal interview.

————, and Merril, Carl R. "Lambda Phage Transcription in Human Fibroblasts." *Virology,* March 1972.

Gelfant, Seymour, and Smith, J. Graham, Jr. "Aging: Noncycling Cells, an Explanation." *Science,* Oct. 27, 1972.

Geriatrics. "Mental Health and Aging: Life Cycle Perspectives." Nov. 1974.

Gershon, David. "Studies on Aging in Nematodes—I. The Nematode as a Model Organism for Aging Research." *Experimental Gerontology,* March 1970.

————. "Detection of Inactive Enzyme Molecules in Ageing Organisms." *Nature,* Sept. 19, 1970.

————, Harriet and David. "Inactive Enzyme Molecules in Aging Mice: Liver Aldolase." *Proceedings of the National Academy of Science,* March 1973.

Glade, Philip R., and Hirschhorn, Kurt. "Products of Lymphoid Cells in Continuous Culture." *American Journal of Pathology,* Vol. 60, 1970.

Glass, H. Bentley. Personal communications.

————. *Science and Ethical Values.* Chapel Hill: University of North Carolina Press, 1965.

————. "Genetics of Aging," in *Aging: Some Social and Biological Aspects.* N. W. Shock, The American Association for the Advancement of Science, 1960.

Goldstein, Allan L. Personal interviews and communications.

————. "The Thymus Gland: Experimental and Clinical Studies of Its Role in the Development and Expression of Immune Functions," in *Advances in Metabolic Disorders,* New York: Vol. 5, Academic Press, 1971.

————, and White, Abraham. "Thymosin and Other Thymic Hormones: Their Nature and Roles in the Thymic Dependency of Immunological

Phenomena," in *Contemporary Topics in Immunology*, New York: Plenum Press, 1973.

————, Cohen, Geraldine H., et al. "Use of Thymosin in the Treatment of Primary Immunodeficiency Diseases and Cancer." Prepublication manuscript.

Goldstein, Samuel. Personal communication.

————. "Biological Aging: An Essentially Normal Process." *Journal of the American Medical Association*, Dec. 23–30, 1974.

————. "Aging In Vitro: Growth of Cultured Cells from the Galapagos Tortoise." *Experimental Cell Research*, Vol. 83, 1974.

————. "The Biology of Aging." *The New England Journal of Medicine*, Nov. 11, 1971.

————, and Moerman, Elena. "Heat-Labile Enzymes in Skin Fibroblasts from Subjects with Progeria." *New England Journal of Medicine*, June 19, 1975.

————, and Moerman, E. J. "Heat-Labile Enzymes in Werner's Syndrome Fibroblasts." *Nature*, May 8, 1975.

————, and Singal, D. P. "Alteration of Fibroblast Gene Products In Vitro from a Subject with Werner's Syndrome." *Nature*, Oct. 25, 1974.

————, and Trieman, G. "Glucose Consumption by Early and Late-Passage Diploid Human Fibroblasts During Growth and Stationary Phase." Prepublication manuscript.

Good, Phillip, and Macieira-Coelho, A. "Ageing Cell Cultures," *Nature* (letter), Nov. 8, 1974.

Gordon, Paul. "Free Radicals and the Aging Process." in *Theoretical Aspects of Aging*. Edited by M. Rockstein, New York: Academic Press, 1974.

Gregoriadis, Gregory. "Enzyme-Carrier Potential of Liposomes in Enzyme Replacement Therapy." *New England Journal of Medicine*, Jan. 23, 1975.

Gruman, Gerald J. Personal communications.

————. "A History of Ideas About the Prolongation of Life: The Evolution of Prolongevity Hypotheses to 1800." *Transactions of the American Philosophical Society*, Dec. 1966.

Guillemin, Roger. Personal communications.

————. "Synthetic Hypothalamic Releasing Factors." Interview in *Reproductive Endocrinology*, 1973.

————, and Burgus, Roger. "The Hormones of the Hypothalamus." *Scientific American*, Nov. 1972.

Gutman, E. "Nervous and Hormonal Mechanisms in the Aging Process." *Experimental Gerontology*, Oct. 1970.

Harman, Denham. Personal interviews and correspondence.

————. "Free Radical Theory of Aging: Effect of Dietary Fat on Discrimination Learning." Presented to American Oil Chemists' Society, 1973.

————. "Statement of Dr. Denham Harman, President, American Aging Association." Before congressional subcommittee hearing testimony on establishing a National Institute on Aging, March 16, 1973.

————. "Free Radical Theory of Aging: Effect of Vitamin E on Tumor Incidence." Presented to Gerontological Society, Puerto Rico, 1972.

————. "Free Radical Theory of Aging: Dietary Implications." *American Journal of Clinical Nutrition,* Aug. 1972.

————. "The Biologic Clock: The Mitochondria?" *Journal of the American Geriatrics Society,* April 1972.

————. "Free Radical Theory of Aging: Effect of the Amount and Degree of Unsaturation of Dietary Fat on Mortality Rate." *Journal of Gerontology,* Vol. 26, No. 4, 1971.

————. "Prolongation of Life: Role of Free Radical Reactions in Aging." *Journal of the American Geriatrics Society,* Aug. 1969.

————. "Free Radical Theory of Aging: Effect of Free Radical Reaction Inhibitors on the Mortality Rate of Male LAF Mice." *Journal of Gerontology,* Oct. 1968.

————. "Atherosclerosis: Possible Ill Effects of the Use of Highly Unsaturated Fats to Lower Serum-Cholesterol Levels." *The Lancet,* Nov. 30, 1957.

————. "How to Live to a Healthy 105." As told to James C. G. Conniff. *Bell Telephone Magazine,* May–June 1969.

Harrington, Alan. *The Immortalist.* New York: Random House, 1969.

Harris, Morgan. *Cell Culture and Somatic Variation.* New York: Holt Rinehart & Winston, 1964.

Harrison, David E. Personal conversations and communications.

————. "Normal Function of Transplanted Marrow Cell Lines from Aged Mice." *Journal of Gerontology,* Vol. 30, No. 3, 1975.

————. "Defective Erythropoietic Responses of Aged Mice Not Improved by Young Marrow." *Journal of Gerontology,* Vol. 30, No. 3, 1975.

————. "Normal Production of Erythrocytes by Mouse Marrow Continuous for 73 Months." *Proceedings of the National Academy of Sciences,* Nov. 1973.

————. "Normal Function of Transplanted Mouse Erythrocyte Precursors for 21 Months Beyond Donor Life Span." *Nature New Biology,* June 16, 1972.

————, and Doubleday, John W. "Normal Function of Immunologic Stem Cells from Aged Mice." *The Journal of Immunology,* April 1975.

Haslam, Richard J., and Goldstein, Samuel. "Adenosine 3':5'–Cyclic

Monophosphate in Young and Senescent Human Fibroblasts during Growth and Stationary Phase In Vitro." *Biochem. J.,* Vol. 144, 1974.

Hayflick, Leonard. Personal interviews and correspondence.

————. "Cell Biology of Aging." *BioScience,* Oct. 1975.

————. "Perspectives in Human Longevity." Presented at Conference on Social Policy, Social Ethics and an Aging Society, University of Chicago, 1975.

————. "Current Theories of Biological Aging." *Federation Proceedings,* Jan. 1975.

————. "Cultured Human Cells and Aging." Presented at American Association for the Advancement of Science, San Francisco, 1974.

————. "The Strategy of Senescence." *The Gerontologist,* Feb. 1974.

————. "The Longevity of Cultured Human Cells." *Journal of the American Geriatrics Society,* Vol. XXII, No. 1, 1974.

————. "Aging Human Cells." *Triangle,* Vol. 12, No. 4, 1973.

————. "The Biology of Human Aging." *American Journal of the Medical Sciences,* Vol. 265, No. 6, 1973.

————. "Cell Senescence and Cell Differentiation In Vitro." in *Altern und Entwicklung.* Stuttgart: F. K. Schattauer Verlag, 1972.

————. "Aging Under Glass." *Experimental Gerontology,* Dec. 1970.

————. "Human Cells and Aging." *Scientific American,* March 1968.

Heinlein, Robert A. *Time Enough for Love.* New York: G. P. Putnam's, 1973.

————. *Methuselah's Children.* New York: New American Library (Signet), 1968.

HEW. Statement of Dr. Charles C. Edwards, Assistant Secretary of Health. Before the Special Committee on Aging. U.S. Senate, Aug. 1, 1974.

HEW News. Release on Robert T. Simpson. Oct. 2, 1974.

Hirokawa, Katsuiku, and Makinodan, T. "Thymic Involution: Effect on T-Cell Differentiation." *Journal of Immunology,* June 1974.

Hirsch, Gerald P., and Strehler, Bernard L. "Cross-tissue Translational Capacities: I. The Adequacy of tRNAs from Heterologous Tissues in the Translation of Hemoglobin Message. II. Relative Effectiveness of Heterologous Synthetases (and Other Supernatant Factors) in the Translation of Hemoglobin Message." *Mechanisms of Ageing and Development,* Vol. 2, 1973.

Hochschild, Richard. Personal communications.

————. "Effect of Dimethylaminoethyl *p*-Chlorophenoxyacetate on the Life Span of Male Swiss Webster Albino Mice." *Experimental Gerontology,* Vol. 8, 1973.

————. "Effect of Dimethylaminoethanol on the Life Span of Senile Male A/J Rats." *Experimental Gerontology,* Vol. 8, 1973.

————. "Effects of Various Drugs on Longevity in Female C57BL/6J Mice." *Gerontologia,* Vol. 19, 1973.

————. "Effects of Various Additives on *In Vitro* Survival Time of Mouse Macrophages." *Journal of Gerontology,* Vol. 28, No. 4, 1973.

————. "Effects of Various Additives on *In Vitro* Survival Time of Human Fibroblasts." *Journal of Gerontology,* Vol. 28, No. 4, 1973.

————. "Lysosomes, Membranes, and Aging." Prepublication manuscript, 1971.

————. "Effects of Membrane Stabilizing Drugs on Mortality in Drosophila Melanogaster." *Experimental Gerontology,* Vol. 6, 1971.

————. "Prospects for the Control of Human Aging." Prepublication manuscript.

Hoehn, Holger, Bryant, Eileen M., et al. "Non-Selective Isolation, Stability and Longevity of Hybrids Between Normal Human Somatic Cells." *Nature,* Dec. 18, 1975.

Hoffman, Jerald L., and McCoy, Martha T. "Stability of the Nucleoside Composition of tRNA during Biological Ageing of Mice and Mosquitoes." *Nature,* June 7, 1974.

Hollander, C. F. "Functional and Cellular Aspects of Organ Ageing." *Experimental Gerontology,* October 1970.

Holliday, Robin. "Errors in Protein Synthesis and Clonal Senescence in Fungi." *Nature,* March 29, 1969.

————, Porterfield, J. S., and Gibbs, D. D. "Premature Ageing and Occurrence of Altered Enzyme in Werner's Syndrome Fibroblasts." *Nature,* Apr. 26, 1974.

Horst, Jürgen, Kluge, Friedrich, et al. "Gene Transfer to Human Cells: Transducing Phage Lambda–p–lac Gene Expression in GM–1 Gangliosidosis Fibroblasts." Prepublication manuscript.

Houston, Jean. "Putting the First Man on Earth." *Saturday Review,* Feb. 22, 1975.

Hruza, Zdanek. Personal communication.

Human Behavior. "Aging." Dec. 1974.

Huyck, Margaret H. *Growing Older.* Englewood Cliffs, N.J.: Prentice-Hall, 1974.

Jacob, François, and Monod, Jacques. "Genetic Regulatory Mechanisms in the Synthesis of Proteins." *Journal of Molecular Biology,* Vol. 3, 1961.

jax. "Sooner or Later, Everyone Begins to Think about Growing Old." Fall 1972.

Johnson, Roger, Chrisp, Clarence, and Strehler, Bernard. "Selective Loss of Ribosomal RNA Genes During the Aging of Post-Mitotic Tissues." *Mechanisms of Ageing and Development,* Vol. 1, 1972.

Juniper, Dean. *Man Against Mortality.* New York: Scribner's, 1973.

Kanungo, M. S. "Biochemistry of Aging." *Biochemical Reviews,* Vol. 41, 1970.

―――, Koul, Omanand, and Reddy, K. R. "Concomitant Studies on RNA Protein Synthesis in Tissues of Rats of Various Ages." *Experimental Gerontology,* Sept. 1970.

Kasten, Frederick H. "Functional Capacity of Neonatal Mammalian Myocardial Cells During Aging in Tissue Culture." Prepublication manuscript.

―――, and Yip, Dominic K. "Reanimation of Cultured Mammalian Myocardial Cells During Multiple Cycles of Trypsinization–Freezing–Thawing." *In Vitro,* Vol. 9, No. 4, 1974.

Kastenbaum, Robert. "Age: Getting There Ahead of Time." *Psychology Today,* Dec. 1971.

Kato, Ryuichi, and Takanaka, Akira. "Metabolism of Drugs in Old Rats." *Japanese Journal of Pharmacology,* Dec. 1968.

Keleman, Stanley. *Living Your Dying.* New York: Random House, 1974.

Kemeny, Gabor, and Rosenberg, Barnett. "Compensation Law in Thermodynamics and Thermal Death." *Nature,* June 15, 1973.

Kishimoto, Susumu, and Yamamura, Yuichi. "Immune Responses in Aged Mice: Changes of Antibody-Forming Cell Precursors and Antigen-Reactive Cells with Ageing." *Clin. exp. Immunol.,* Vol. 8, 1971.

―――, Shigemoto, Shozo, and Yamamura, Yuichi. "Immune Response in Aged Mice: Change of Cell-Mediated Immunity with Ageing." *Transplantation,* Vol. 15, No. 5, 1973.

Klebe, Robert J., Chen, Tchaw-Ren, and Ruddle, Frank H. "Controlled Production of Proliferating Somatic Cell Hybrids." *Journal of Cell Biology,* Vol. 45, 1970.

Klemme, Herbert. "The Later Years—Are You Ready?" *Menninger Perspective,* Fall 1974.

Kohn, Robert R. Personal conversation.

―――. *Principles of Mammalian Aging.* Englewood Cliffs, N.J.: Prentice-Hall, 1971.

―――. "Aging and Cell Division." *Science* (letter), Apr. 18, 1975.

―――. "Principles of Mammalian Aging." Presentation to American Association for the Advancement of Science, San Francisco, 1974.

Konigsmark, Bruce W., and Murphy, Edmond A. "Neuronal Populations in the Human Brain." *Nature,* Dec. 26, 1970.

Kormendy, Charles G., and Bender, A. Douglas. "Chemical Interference with Aging." *Gerontologia,* 1971.

―――. "Experimental Modification of the Chemistry and Biology of the Aging Process." *Journal of Pharmaceutical Science,* Feb. 1971.

Krohn, P. L. "Review Lectures on Senescence. II: Heterochronic

Transplantation in the Study of Ageing." *Proceedings of the Royal Society,* Vol. 157, Dec. 18, 1962.

Laboratory Management. "Regenerating the Heart Muscle Cell." Aug. 1973.

Lambert, Darwin. "Bristlecone Harmonies." *National Parks & Conservation Magazine,* March 1972.

The Lancet. "Thymus Hormones" (editorial). Feb. 8, 1975.

Lang, Calvin A., "Biological Age. A Key Parameter in Aging Research," presented at AAAs meeting, San Francisco, 1974.

————. "Macromolecular Changes During the Life-Span of the Mosquito." *Journal of Gerontology,* Oct. 1967.

Lansing, A. I. "A Transmissible, Cumulative and Reversible Factor in Aging." *Journal of Gerontology,* Vol. 2, No. 3, 1974.

Lappé, Marc and Morrison, Robert S., *Ethical and Scientific Issues Posed by Human Uses of Molecular Genetics,* New York Academy of Sciences, 1976.

Lazarus, Gerald S. "Mechanisms of Connective Tissue Degradation." *Science,* Nov. 15, 1974.

Leaf, Alexander. *Youth in Old Age.* New York: McGraw-Hill, 1975.

————. "Unusual Longevity: The Common Denominators." *Hospital Practice,* Oct. 1973.

————. "The Peaks of Old Age." *Observer Magazine,* Sept. 30, 1973.

————. "Where Life Begins at 100." *National Geographic,* Jan. 1973.

Lederberg, Joshua. "Biomedical Frontiers: Genetics," in *The Challenge of Life* (Roche Anniversary Symposium), Basel, Switzerland: Birkäuser Verlag, 1972.

————. "Biomedical Research: Its Side-Effects and Challenges." *Stanford MD,* Oct. 1967.

————. "Experimental Genetics and Human Evolution." *Bulletin of the Atomic Scientists,* Oct. 1966.

————. "Biological Future of Man," in *Man and His Future,* edited by Gordon Wolstenholme, a Ciba symposium. Boston: Little Brown, 1963.

Lee, Catherine T., and Duerre, John A. "Changes in Histone Methylase Activity of Rat Brain and Liver with Ageing." *Nature,* Sept. 20, 1974.

Lehman, Harvey C. *Age and Achievement.* Princeton: Princeton University Press, 1953.

Lehninger, Albert L. "How Cells Transform Energy." *Scientific American,* Sept. 1961.

Leonard, George. *The Transformation.* New York: Dell Publishing Co., 1972.

Leopold, A. C. "Aging, Senescence and Turnover in Plants." *BioScience,* Oct. 1975.

Levine, Ghita. "Trying to Slow Down Aging." *Baltimore Sunday Sun,* July 16, 1972.

Lewin, Roger. *Hormones: Chemical Communicators.* Garden City, N.Y.: Doubleday Anchor Press, 1973.

Lifton, Robert Jay. "The Sense of Immortality: On Death and the Continuity of Life," in *Explorations in Psychohistory.* New York: Simon & Schuster, 1974.

Liu, R. K., and Walford, R. L. "The Effect of Lowered Body Temperature on Lifespan and Immune and Non-Immune Processes." *Gerontologia,* Vol. 18, 1972.

————. "Observations on the Lifespans of Several Species of Annual Fishes and the World's Smallest Fishes." *Experimental Gerontology,* Sept. 1970.

Loeb, J., and Northrop, J. H. "Is There a Temperature Coefficient for the Duration of Life?" *Proceedings of the National Academy of Sciences,* Vol. 2, 1916.

————. "On the Influence of Food and Temperature upon the Duration of Life." *Journal of Biological Chemistry,* Vol. 32, No. 1, 1917.

Ludwig, Frederic. Personal communication.

Lunzer, Steven. Personal conversations.

————. "Aging: Causes and Treatment." Unpublished manuscript.

Luria, S. E. *Life—The Unfinished Experiment.* New York: Scribner's, 1973.

————. "Ethical Aspects of the New Perspectives in Biomedical Research," in *The Challenge of Life* (Roche Anniversary Symposium). Basel, Switzerland: Birkhäuser Verlag, 1972.

Macieira-Coelho, A., and Loria, E. "Stimulation of Ribosome Synthesis During Retarded Ageing of Human Fibroblasts by Hydrocortisone." *Nature,* Sept. 6, 1974.

Maisel, Albert Q. "The 'Useless' Gland That Guards Our Health." *Reader's Digest,* Nov. 1966.

————. "Can Science Prolong Our Useful Years?" *Reader's Digest,* Jan. 1962.

Makinodan, T., and Adler, W. H. "The Effects of Aging on the Differentiation and Proliferation Potentials of Cells of the Immune System." Prepublication manuscript for *Federation Proceedings,* 1974.

Martin, George M., Sprague, Curtis A., and Epstein, Charles J. "Replicative Life-Span of Cultivated Human Cells: Effects of Donor's Age, Tissue, and Genotype." *Laboratory Investigation,* Vol. 23, No. 1, 1970.

Martin, George M., Sprague, Curtis A., et al. "Clonal Selection, Attenuation, and Differentiation in an In Vitro Model of Hyperplasia." *American Journal of Pathology,* Jan. 1974.

Marx, Jean L. "Suppressor T Cells: Role in Immune Regulation." *Science,* Apr. 18, 1975.

———. "T Cell Maturation." *Science,* Mar. 28, 1975.

———. "Aging Research (I): Cellular Theories of Senescence." *Science,* Dec. 20, 1974.

———. "Aging Research (II): Pacemakers for Aging?" *Science,* Dec. 27, 1974.

Massachusetts Institute of Technology. News release on Har Gobind Khorana, Sept. 11, 1974.

Masters, William H. "Sex Steroid Influences on the Aging Process." *American Journal of Obstetrics and Gynecology,* Oct. 1957.

Mathews, J. D., Whittingham, S., and Mackay, I. R. "Autoimmune Mechanisms in Human Vascular Disease." *The Lancet,* Dec. 14, 1974.

McBride, Gail. "Gene-grafting Experiments Produce both High Hopes and Grave Worries." A two-part article in "Medical News" sections of *Journal of the American Medical Association,* Apr. 28 and May 5, 1975.

McCay, Clive M., Maynard, L. A., et al. "Retarded Growth, Life Span, Ultimate Body Size and Age Changes in the Albino Rat after Feeding Diets Restricted in Calories." *Journal of Nutrition,* Vol. 18, 1939.

McGrady, Patrick M., Jr. *The Youth Doctors.* New York: Coward-McCann, Inc., 1968.

McMahon, Daniel. "Chemical Messengers in Development: A Hypothesis." *Science,* Sept. 20, 1974.

McQuade, Walter. "What Stress Can Do to You." *Fortune,* Jan. 1972.

Mead, James F. "Polyunsaturated Fatty Acids." *Science,* June 20, 1975.

Meadow, Norman D., and Barrow, Charles H., Jr. "Studies on Aging in a Bdelloid Rotifer. II. The Effects of Various Environmental Conditions and Maternal Age on Longevity and Fecundity." *Journal of Gerontology,* Vol. 26, No. 3, 1971.

———. "Studies on Aging in a Bdelloid Rotifer." *The Journal of Experimental Zoology,* March 1971.

Medawar, Peter B. *The Future of Man.* New York: Mentor Books, 1959.

———. *Aging: An Unsolved Problem of Biology.* London: H. K. Lewis, 1952.

———. "Life in the Deep Freeze." *New York Times,* Sept. 6, 1973.

———. "The Growth-Energy and Ageing of the Chicken's Heart." *Proceedings of the Royal Society,* Vol. B129, 1940.

Medical Tribune. "Aging Linked to Decrease in Thymosin Blood Levels." June 13, 1973.

———. "First Thymosin Clinical Trials Show Promise." Sept. 4, 1974.

Medical World News. "Synthesizing Against Senility." June 28, 1974.

———. "Bringing Research on Aging Up to Date." Apr. 19, 1974.

————. "Amyloid—Aging Link Gets Support." Nov. 9, 1973.

————. "Giant Step in Genetic Engineering." Oct. 5, 1973.

————. "Human Genetic Engineering." May 11, 1973.

————. "Aging: Investigators Probe Biochemical, Genetic Aspects of Universal 'Disease.' " Oct. 22, 1971.

Medvedev, Zhores A. Personal interview and communications.

————. *Protein Biosynthesis and Problems of Heredity, Development, and Ageing.* Edinburgh: Oliver & Boyd, 1966.

————. "Ageing and Lifespan." A Royal Institution lecture, London, 1973.

————. "Possible Role of Repeated Nucleotide Sequences in DNA in the Evolution of Life Spans of Differentiated Cells." *Nature,* June 23, 1973.

Merril, Carl R. Personal interviews and communications.

————. "Interactions of Bacterial Viruses and Bacterial Genes with Animal Systems." Prepublication manuscript.

————, Geier, Mark R., and Rolfe, Barry G. "Characteristics of Bacterial Gene Expression in Human Fibroblasts." Prepublication manuscript.

————, and Petricciani, John C. "Bacterial Virus Gene Expression in Human Cells." *Nature,* Oct. 8, 1971.

Miller, J. F. A. P. "Endocrine Function of the Thymus." *New England Journal of Medicine,* May 30, 1974.

Miquel, Jaime. "Morphological Changes in the Aging Drosophila Melanogaster." Presented at American Association for the Advancement of Science, San Francisco, 1974.

————. Bensch, Klaus G., et al. "Natural Aging and Radiation-Induced Life Shortening in Drosophila Melanogaster." *Mechanisms of Ageing and Development,* Vol. 1, 1972.

Moment, Gairdner. "The Ponce de Leon Trail Today." *BioScience,* Oct. 1975.

Monod, Jacques. *Chance and Necessity.* New York: Alfred A. Knopf, 1971.

Muggleton, Audrey, and Danielli, J. F. "Inheritance of the 'Life-Spanning' Phenomenon in *Amoeba proteus.*" *Experimental Cell Research,* Vol. 49, 1968.

Munro, A. J., and Taussig, M. J. "Two genes in the Major Histocompatibility Complex Control Immune Response." *Nature,* July 10, 1975.

Nandy, Kalidas. Personal communications.

————. "Further Studies on the Effects of Centrophenoxine on the Lipofuscin Pigment in the Neurons of Senile Guinea Pigs." *Journal of Gerontology,* Jan. 1968.

Nature. "Transduction of Human Cells by Lambda" (editorial). Oct. 8, 1971.

Neugarten, Bernice L. "Social Implications of a Prolonged Life-Span." *The Gerontologist,* Winter 1972.

————. "Age: Grow Old Along With Me! The Best Is Yet To Be." *Psychology Today,* Dec. 1971.

New Scientist. "What's the Value of Thinking about Ageing?" Sept. 13, 1973.

————. "Ageing: Is It Nature's Intent Rather than Error?" May 10, 1972.

Newsweek. "Can Aging Be Cured?" April 16, 1973.

Niewiarowski, Stefan, and Goldstein, Samuel. "Interaction of Cultured Human Fibroblasts with Fibrin: Modification by Drugs and Aging In Vitro." *Journal of Laboratory and Clinical Medicine,* Oct. 1973.

Nikitin, V. N. "The Genetic Apparatus and Aging Processes," in *The Main Problems of Soviet Gerontology,* Kiev, 1972.

Nirenberg, Marshall W. "The Genetic Code: II." *Scientific American,* March 1963.

Northrop, J. "The Effect of Prolongation of the Period of Growth on the Total Duration of Life." *Journal of Biological Chemistry,* Vol. 32, 1917.

Norwood, Thomas H. Personal communication.

————, Pendergrass, William R., et al. "Dominance of the Senescent Phenotype in Heterokaryons Between Replicative and Post-Replicative Human Fibroblast-Like Cells." *Proceedings of the National Academy of Sciences,* June 1974.

Orgel, Leslie E. Personal communications.

————. "Ageing of Clones of Mammalian Cells." *Nature,* June 22, 1973.

Otto, A. Stuart. Personal communications.

————. Editorials in *The Immortality Newsletter.*

Packer, Lester. Personal communication.

————, and Smith, James R. "Extension of the Lifespan of Cultured Normal Human Diploid Cells by Vitamin E." Prepublication manuscript.

Passwater, Richard A. Personal communications.

————. "Cancer: New Directions." *American Laboratory,* June 1973.

————. "Dietary Cholesterol: Is It Related to Serum Cholesterol and Heart Disease?" *American Laboratory,* Sept. 1972.

————, and Welker, Paul A. "Human Aging Research." A two-part article, *American Laboratory,* April and May, 1971.

Patrusky, Ben. "Of Mice and Men—and the Aging Factor." *Signature,* Jan. 1971.

Patton, Stuart, and Trams, Eberhard G. "Salmon Heart Triglycerides During Spawning Migration." *Comp. Biochem. Physiol.,* Vol. 46B, 1973.

Pecile, A., Müller, E., and Falconi, G. "Endocrine Function of Pituitary Transplants Taken from Rats of Different Ages." *Arch. Int. Pharmacodyn.,* Vol. 2, 1966.

Pelc, S. R. "Metabolic DNA and the Problem of Ageing." *Experimental Gerontology,* Sept. 1970.

Peng, Ming-tsung, and Huang, Hive-ho. "Aging of Hypothalamic-Pituitary-Ovarian Function in the Rat." *Fertility and Sterility,* Aug. 1972.

Petes, T. D., Farber, R. A., et al. "Altered Rate of DNA Replication in Ageing Human Fibroblast Cultures." *Nature,* Oct. 4, 1974.

Platt, Dieter. Personal communication.

————, Hering, H., and Hering, F. J. "Age Dependent Determination of Lysosomal Enzyme Activities in the Liver and Brain as Well as the Measurements of Cytoplasmic Enzyme Activities in the Blood of Piracetam Pre-Treated Rats." Experimental Gerontology, Vol. 8, 1973.

————, and Pauli, H. "Effect of Alpha-Napthylisothiocyanate on Lysosomal Enzymes and 14C-Leucine-Incorporation of Liver and Spleen of Young and Old Rats." *Actuelle Gerontologie,* July 1972.

————. "Age Dependent Determinations of Lysosomal Enzymes in the Liver of Spironolactone and Aldosterone Pretreated Rats." Experimental Gerontology, Vol. 7, 1972.

Prehoda, Robert W. *Extended Youth.* New York: G. P. Putnam's, 1968.

————. "Retardation of Aging." *Medical Opinion & Review,* Oct. 1970.

Price, Gerald B., Modak, S. P., and Makinodan, P. "Age-Associated Changes in the DNA of Mouse Tissue." *Science,* March 5, 1971.

Public Law 93–296, 93rd Congress, S. 775, "An Act to amend the Public Health Service Act to provide for the establishment of a National Institute on Aging," May 31, 1974.

Pythilä, M. J., and Sinex, F. Marott. "The Effect of Diet on the Composition of Chromatin from Young and Old Rats." *Experimental Gerontology,* March 1970.

Quadri, S. K., Kledzik, G. S., and Meites, J. "Reinitiation of Estrous Cycles in Old Constant-Estrous Rats by Central-Acting Drugs." *Neuroendocrinology,* Vol. 11, 1973.

Ratcliff, J. D. "I Am Joe's Thyroid," *Reader's Digest,* March 1973.

————. "I Am Joe's Pituitary Gland." *Reader's Digest,* Nov. 1972.

————. "I Am Joe's Hypothalamus." *Reader's Digest,* March 1970.

————. "Your Amazing Glands." *Family Doctor,* Nov. 1958.

Reichel, William. Personal interviews and communications.

————. "Premature Aging." Presented at 9th International Congress of Gerontology, Kiev, 1972.

————. "The Biology of Aging." *Journal of the American Geriatrics Society,* Vol. 14, 1966.

————. "Lipofuscin Pigment Accumulation in Five Rat Organs as a Function of Age." *Journal of Gerontology,* Apr. 1968.

————, Hollander, Joshua, et al. "Lipofuscin Pigment Accumulation as a Function of Age and Distribution in Rodent Brain." *Journal of Gerontology,* Jan. 1968.

————, Bailey, Joseph A., et al. "Radiological Findings in Progeria." *Journal of the American Geriatrics Society,* Aug. 1971.

————, Garcia-Bunuel, Rafael, and DiLallo, Joseph. "Progeria and Werner's Syndrome as Models for the Study of Normal Human Aging." *Journal of the American Geriatrics Society,* May 1971.

Riggs, A. D. "How Genes Are Regulated." *City of Hope Quarterly,* Summer 1975.

Robert, L., Robert, B., and Robert, A. M. "Molecular Biology of Elastin as Related to Aging and Atherosclerosis." *Experimental Gerontology,* Oct. 1970.

Robertson, Miranda. "ICI Puts Money on Genetic Engineering." *Nature,* Oct. 18, 1974.

Roberts-Thomson, Ian C., Whittingham, S., et al. "Ageing, Immune Response, and Mortality." *The Lancet,* Aug. 17, 1974.

Robinson, Arthur B., McKerrow, James H., and Cary, Paul. "Controlled Deamination of Peptides and Proteins: An Experimental Hazard and a Possible Biological Timer." *Proceedings of the National Academy of Sciences,* July 1970.

Rockstein, Morris, ed. *Theoretical Aspects of Aging.* New York: Academic Press, 1974.

————, and Hawkins, W. Brown. "Thiamine in the Ageing House Fly, *Musca domestica.*" *Experimental Gerontology,* July 1970.

Rodgers, Joann. "Genetic Engineering Poses Danger to Mankind." *Baltimore News American,* Aug. 18, 1974.

Rolfe, Barry G. Personal communications.

————. "Phage-Mediated Transgenosis in Human Fibroblasts." Prepublication manuscript.

Rosenberg, Barnett. Personal communications.

————, Kemeny, Gabor, et al. "The Kinetics and Thermodynamics of Death in Multicellular Organisms." *Mechanisms of Ageing and Development,* Vol. 2, 1973.

————. "Quantitative Evidence for Protein Denaturation as the Cause of Thermal Death." *Nature,* Aug. 13, 1971.

Rosenfeld, Albert. *The Second Genesis: The Coming Control of Life.* Englewood Cliffs, N.J.: Prentice-Hall, 1969; New York: Vintage paperback, Random House, 1975.

———. "The Death of Old Age?" *Nature/Science Annual.* New York: Time-Life Books, 1975.

———. "The Conquest of Old Age." CBS-TV "Summer Semester," July 11, 1975.

———. "Thymosin: Breaking the Immune Barrier." *Saturday Review,* June 15, 1974.

———. "The Longevity Seekers." *Saturday Review of the Sciences,* March 1973.

———, ed. "Mind and Supermind: Expanding the Limits of Consciousness." Special section in *Saturday Review,* Feb. 22, 1975.

———, and Hills, Alicia. "DNA's Code: Key to All Life." *Life,* Oct. 4, 1963.

Rostand, Jean. *Humanly Possible.* New York: Saturday Review Press, 1973.

———. *Can Man Be Modified?* New York: Basic Books, 1959.

Rostovsky, Igor L. "Aging: Oceanography and Geriatrics." *Oceans,* Feb. 1969.

Rous, Peyton. "Presentation of the Kober Medal for 1961 to O. H. Robertson." *Transactions of the American Association of Physicians,* 1961.

Ruddle, Frank H. "Cell Fusion as a Tool in the Study of Cellular Biology." Presented at National Foundation–March of Dimes conference, Harbor Springs, Mich., 1975.

———. "Linkage Analysis in Man by Somatic Cell Genetics." *Nature,* March 16, 1973.

———, and Kucherlapati, Raju S. "Hybrid Cells and Human Genes." *Scientific American,* July 1974.

Ruiz-Carillo, Adolfo, Wangh, Lawrence J., and Allfrey, Vincent G. "Processing of Newly Synthesized Histone Molecules." *Science,* Oct. 10, 1975.

Russell, Elizabeth S. Personal communications.

Sacher, George A. "The Evolutionary-Genetic Approach to Mammalian Longevity and Aging." Presented at American Association for the Advancement of Science, San Francisco, 1974.

Sacktor, Bertram, and Shimada, Yoshio. "Degenerative Changes in the Mitochondria of Flight Muscle from Aging Blowflies." *Journal of Cell Biology,* Vol. 52, 1972.

Salk, Jonas. Personal communications.

———. *The Survival of the Wisest.* New York: Harper & Row, 1973.

Salk Institute Newsletter. "Study on Aging Reported by Dr. Orgel." No. 5, Fall 1973.

Sanadi, D. Rao. Personal interview and communications.

———, Chen, J. C., and Warshaw, J. B. "Decline of Mitochondrial

Respiration in Senescence." Presented at International Study Group for Research in Cardiac Metabolism, Winnipeg, 1972.

Sanders, Howard J. "Human Aging: the Enigma Persists." *Chemical & Engineering News,* July 24, 1972.

Sarkar, Bibudhendra. "Design of Active Site Substitutes." *Guidelines to Metabolic Therapy,* Spring 1975.

Scheinberg, Morton A., Goldstein, Allan L., and Cathcart, Edgar S. "Thymosin Restores T Cell Function and Reduces the Incidence of Amyloid Disease in Casein-Treated Mice." *Journal of Immunology,* Jan. 1976.

————, Cathcart, Edgar S., and Goldstein, Allan L. "Thymosin-Induced Reduction of 'Null Cells' in Peripheral-Blood Lymphocytes of Patients with Systemic Lupus Erythematosus." *The Lancet,* Feb. 22, 1975.

Schloss, Benjamin. Personal interviews and communications.

————. "The Control of Human Aging" (mimeographed). Foundation for Aging Research, Los Angeles, 1974.

————. "Breaking Man's Lifespan Barrier" (mimeographed). Foundation for Aging Research, Los Angeles, 1974.

————. *Prolonging Youthfulness* (brochure). Foundation for Aging Research, Brooklyn, N.Y., 1970.

————. "Can Fundamental Discoveries in Complex Biological Systems Be Programmed?" Prepublication manuscript.

————. "A Theory of Matter/Its Application to Aging." Prepublication manuscript.

Schmeck, Harold M. *Immunology: The Many-Edged Sword.* New York: George Braziller, 1974.

————. "Researchers Discover Method of Transferring Cell Nuclei in Living Tissue." *New York Times,* June 17, 1974.

————. "Human Cells in Test Use Genetic Matter Native to Bacteria." *New York Times,* Oct. 14, 1971.

————. "Science: Extending the Life Span." *New York Times,* May 30, 1965.

Schmid, Rudolf and Schmid, Marvin J. "Living Links with the Past." *Natural History,* March 1975.

The Sciences. "Slowing the Biological Clock." July 1970.

Segall, Paul E., and Timiras, Paola S. "Age-related changes in thermoregulatory capacity of tryptophan-deficient rats." *Federation Proceedings,* Jan. 1975.

————. "Reproductive and Behavioral Effects of Aging Retardation." Prepublication manuscript.

————, and Waitz, Harold D. "Long Term Tryptophan Deficiency and Aging Retardation in the Rat." Prepublication report.

————, Miller, C., and Timiras, P. S. "Aging and CNS Monoamines."
Prepublication report.

Segerberg, Osborn, Jr. *The Immortality Factor.* New York: E. P. Dutton,
1974.

Shaw, George Bernard. *Back to Methuselah,* in *Complete Plays with
Prefaces,* Vol. II. New York: Dodd, Mead, 1963.

Shefer, V. F. "Absolute Number of Neurons and Thickness of the
Cerebral Cortex During Aging, Senile and Vascular Dementia, and
Pick's and Alzheimer's Diseases." *Zhurnal Nevropatologii i Psikhiatrii
imeni S.S. Korsokava,* Vol. 72, No. 7, 1972.

Sheldrake, A. R. "The Ageing, Growth and Death of Cells." *Nature,*
Aug. 2, 1974.

Shock, Nathan W. "Will You Live to Be 100?" *Britannica Yearbook,*
1972.

————. "Physiologic Aspects of Aging." *Journal of the American
Dietetic Association,* June 1970.

————. "The Physiology of Aging." *Scientific American,* Jan. 1962.

————. "The Physiology of Aging," book chapter. GRC/Baltimore.

Shurkin, Joel N. "Scientists Belittle Hopes of Living Beyond 90 Years."
Philadelphia Inquirer, March 2, 1974.

Siakotos, A. N., and Armstrong, Donald. "Age Pigment, A Biochemical
Indicator of Intracellular Aging," in *Neurobiology of Aging.* Edited
by J. M. Ordy and K. R. Brizzee. New York: Plenum Publishing Co.,
1975.

Sinex, F. Marott. Personal interviews and communications.

————. "The Molecular Genetics of Aging." Prepublication manuscript.

————. Testimony before congressional subcommittee on aging-research needs, 1971.

————. "Genetic Mechanisms of Aging." *Journal of Gerontology,* July
1966.

Smith, James R. Personal communication.

Smith, John Maynard. Personal communication.

————. "Molecular Evolution and the Age of Man." *Nature,* Feb. 13,
1975.

————. "Review Lectures on Senescence I: The Causes of Ageing."
Proceedings of the Royal Society, Vol. 157, Dec. 18, 1962.

————. "A Theory of Ageing." *Nature,* Vol. 184, 1959.

————, Boscuk, A. N., and Tebbutt, Susan. "Protein Turnover in
Adult Drosophila." *Journal of Insect Physiology,* Vol. 16, 1970.

Sonneborn, Tracy M., ed. *The Control of Human Heredity and Evolution.* New York: Macmillan, 1965.

Srivastava, Satish K. Personal interviews and communications.

————. "Antibody Against Purified Human Hexosaminidase B Cross-

Reacting with Human Hexosaminidase A." *Biochemical and Biophysical Research Communications,* May 26, 1972.

————, and Beutler, E. "Hexosaminidase-A and Hexosaminidase-B: Studies in Tay-Sachs and Sandhoff's Disease." *Nature,* Feb. 16, 1973.

————, Awasthi, Yogesh C., et al. "Studies on Human beta-D-N-Acetylhexosaminidases. I. Purification and Properties. II. Kinetic and Structural Properties. III. Biochemical Genetics of Tay-Sachs and Sandhoff's Disease" (three articles). *Journal of Biological Chemistry,* Apr. 10, 1974.

Stanley, Jean F., Pye, David, and MacGregor, Andrew. "Comparison of Doubling Numbers Attained by Cultured Animal Cells with Life Span of Species." *Nature,* May 8, 1975.

Stein, Gary S., Stein, Janet Swinehart, and Kleinsmith, Lewis J. "Chromosomal Proteins and Gene Regulation." *Scientific American,* Feb. 1975.

Steward, F. C. "Cloning Cells and Controlling the Composition of Crops." *Progress: The Unilever Quarterly,* No. 2, 1970.

————. "Totipotency, Variation and Clonal Development of Cultured Cells." *Endeavour,* Sept. 1970.

Stewart, Fred Mustard. *The Methuselah Enzyme.* New York: Arbor House, 1970.

Strehler, Bernard L. Personal interviews and communications.

————. *Time, Cells, and Aging.* New York: Academic Press, 1962.

————. "How to Stay Young." Prepublication manuscript.

————. "Aging: Transcriptional and Translational Control Mechanisms and Their Alteration." Presented at American Association for the Advancement of Science, San Francisco, 1974.

————. "Implications of Aging Research for Society." Presented at Federation of American Societies for Experimental Biology, Atlantic City, N.J., 1974.

————. "A New Age for Aging." *Natural History,* Feb. 1973.

————. "Lengthening Our Lives." *Science Yearbook,* 1973.

————. Testimony before congressional subcommittees on aging-research needs, 1967, 1971, and 1972.

————. "Men, Molecules and Mortality: Effects of Life Extension." Presented at Council for the Advancement of Science Writing, Boulder, Colo., 1972.

————. "Synopsis of an Engram Storage, Retrieval and Manipulation System: A Parsimonious Model for Higher Brain Function." Prepublication manuscript, 1972.

————. "Aging at the Cellular Level," in *Clinical Geriatrics.* Edited by Isadore Rossman. Philadelphia: J. B. Lippincott, 1971.

————. "Ten Myths About Aging." *Center Magazine,* July 1970.

————. "Information Handling in the Nervous System: An Analogy to Molecular-Genetic Coder-Decoder Mechanisms." *Perspectives in Biology and Medicine,* Summer 1969.

————. "The Prometheus Experiment." *Perspectives in Biology and Medicine,* Winter 1968.

————. "Environmental Factors in Aging and Mortality." *Environmental Research,* Vol. 1, 1967.

————. "Origin and Comparison of the Effects of Time and High-Energy Radiations on Living Systems. *Quarterly Review of Biology,* Vol. 34, No. 2, 1959.

————. "Immortality," in *Science and the Future.* Science Clubs of America, Washington, 1943.

————, Hirsch, G., et al. "Codon-restriction Theory of Aging and Development." *Journal of Theoretical Biology,* Vol. 33, 1971.

————, and Mildvan, A. S. "General Theory of Mortality and Aging." *Science,* Vol. 132, 1960.

————. "Studies on the Chemical Properties of Lipofuscin Age Pigments." Prepublication paper for proceedings of the 5th International Gerontological Congress.

Stuart, Friend. *How to Conquer Physical Death.* San Marcos, Calif.: Dominion Press, 1968.

Stumpf, Samuel E. "Genetic Engineering." *Vanderbilt Alumnus,* Summer 1975.

————. "The Expanding New World of Second-Story People." Presented at American Association for the Advancement of Science, Chicago, 1959.

Stumpf, Walter E. Personal communication.

————, and Sar, Madhabananda. "Localization of Thyroid Hormone in the Mature Rat Brain and Pituitary." *Anatomical Neuroendocrinology.* Prepublication manuscript.

————, and Grant, Lester D. "The Brain: An Endocrine Organ and Hormone Target." *Science,* Dec. 20, 1974.

Sullivan, Jerome L., and DeBusk, A. Gib. "Inositol-less Death in *Neurospora* and Cellular Aging." *Nature New Biology,* May 16, 1973.

Sullivan, Walter. "Scientists Seek Key to Longevity." *New York Times,* Feb. 11, 1973.

————. "Aging: The Eternal Quest for Eternal Youth." *New York Times,* Oct. 24, 1971.

————. "Scientist Foresees a Longer Life Span, Mainly for the Affluent." *New York Times,* Feb. 23, 1971.

————. "Medicine: The Mystery of Aging." *New York Times,* Oct. 30, 1966.

Swan, Henry. Personal communications.

————. "Metabolic Torpor in *Protopterus aethiopicus:* An Anti-Metabolic Agent from the Brain." *American Naturalist,* May–June, 1969.

Szilard, Leo. "On the Nature of the Aging Process." *Proceedings of the National Academy of Sciences,* Vol. 45, 1959.

————. "A Theory of Ageing." *Nature,* Vol. 184, 1959.

Talbert, George B., and Krohn, P. L. "Effect of Maternal Age on Viability of Ova and Uterine Support of Pregnancy in Mice." *J. Reprod. Fert.,* Vol. 11, 1966.

Tappel, A. L. "Will Antitoxidant Nutrients Slow Aging Processes?" *Geriatrics,* Oct. 1968.

————. "Where Old Age Begins." *Nutrition Today,* Dec. 1967.

Tata, J. R. "How Specific Are Nuclear 'Receptors' for Thyroid Hormones?" *Nature,* Sept. 4, 1975.

Taub, Harold J. "Is It True What They Say About Ginseng?" *Let's Live,* June 1975.

Thomas, Lewis. *The Lives of a Cell.* New York: Viking Press, 1974.

————. "The Future Impact of Science and Technology on Medicine." American College of Surgeons *Bulletin,* June 1974.

Time. "Americans Can—and Should—Live Longer." July 10, 1972.

————. "Transplanting a Gene." Oct. 25, 1971.

————. "The Old in the Country of the Young." Aug. 3, 1970.

————. "The Problem of Old Age: Adding Life to Years." July 23, 1956.

Timiras, Paola. Personal communication.

————. "Neurophysiological Factors in Aging: Recent Advances." Presented at International Congress of Gerontology, Jerusalem, 1975.

————. "Aging of Homeostatic Control Systems: Introductory Remarks." *Federation Proceedings,* Jan. 1975.

Toffler, Alvin. *Future Shock.* New York: Random House, 1970.

Tomasch, Joseph. "Comments on 'Neuromythology.' " *Nature,* Sept. 3, 1971.

Trams, Eberhard G. Personal communication.

————. "Hepatic Insufficiency in Spawning Pacific Salmon." *Marine Biology,* Sept. 1969.

————. "Neurochemical Observations on Spawning Pacific Salmon." *Nature,* May 3, 1969.

Travis, Dorothy. Personal conversation.

Treffers, Henry P., Spinelli, Viola, and Belser, Nao O. "A Factor (or Mutator Gene) Influencing Mutation Rates in *Escherichia coli.*" *Proceedings of the National Academy of Sciences,* Vol. 40, 1954.

Trigg, Michael E., Geier, Mark R., et al. "Addition of Leucine Precursors to the Diet of Leucine-Starved Mice." Prepublication manuscript.

Tumbleson, Mike. Personal communications.

Tuccille, Jerome. *Here Comes Immortality,* Stein & Day, New York, 1974.

Turner, Michael D. "Carcinoembryonic Antigen." *Journal of the American Medical Association,* Feb. 17, 1975.

Ubell, Earl. *How to Save Your Life.* New York: Harcourt Brace Jovanovich, 1973.

Unamuno, Miguel de. *The Tragic Sense of Life.* New York: Dover Publications, 1954.

Vaisrub, Samuel. "Nature's Experiment in Unnatural Aging." *Journal of the American Medical Association,* Dec. 24–31, 1973.

Van den Bosch, F. J. G. Personal conversations.

Villee, Dorothy B., Nichols, George, Jr., and Talbot, Nathan B. "Metabolic Studies in Two Boys with Classical Progeria." *Pediatrics,* Feb. 1969.

von Hahn, Holger P. "The Regulation of Protein Synthesis in the Ageing Cell." *Experimental Gerontology,* Oct. 1970.

Walford, Roy L. Personal interview and communications.

———. *The Immunologic Theory of Aging.* Baltimore: Williams & Wilkins, 1969.

———. "The Immunologic Theory of Aging: Current Status." *Federation Proceedings,* 1973.

———. "Introduction" (section on immune dysfunction and aging). *Gerontologia,* Vol. 18, No. 5–6, 1972.

———. Testimony before congressional subcommittee on aging-research needs, 1972.

Wara, Diane W., Goldstein, Allan L., et al. "Thymosin Activity in Patients with Cellular Immunodeficiency." *New England Journal of Medicine,* Jan. 9, 1975.

Watson, James D. *The Molecular Biology of the Gene.* New York: W. A. Benjamin, 1970.

———, and Crick, Francis H. C. "A Structure for Deoxyribose Nucleic Acid." *Nature,* Apr. 25, 1953.

Webb, J. N. "Muscular Dystrophy and Muscle Cell Death in Normal Foetal Development." *Nature,* Nov. 15, 1974.

Weglicki, William B., Reichel, William, and Nair, Padmanabhan P. "Accumulation of Lipofuscin-Like Pigment in the Rat Adrenal Gland as a Function of Vitamin E Deficiency." *Journal of Gerontology,* Oct. 1968.

Weinbach, E. C. "Oxidative Phosphorylation in Mitochondria from Aged Rats." *Journal of Biological Chemistry,* Vol. 234, 1959.

Weissmann, Gerald. Personal conversations.

———. "Enzyme Replacement Therapy." Presented at Council for the Advancement of Science Writing, Ann Arbor, Mich., 1975.

————, Bloomgarden, David, et al. "A General Method for the Introduction of Enzymes, by Means of Immunoglobulin-Coated Liposomes, into Lysosomes of Deficient Cells." *Proceedings of the National Academy of Sciences,* January 1975.

West, C. E., and Redgrave, T. G. "Reservations on the Use of Polyunsaturated Fats in Human Nutrition." *Search,* March 1974.

Wheeler, K. T., and Lett, J. T. "On the Possibility That DNA Repair is Related to Age in Non-Dividing Cells." *Proceedings of the National Academy of Science,* May 1974.

White, Abraham. Personal conversations and communications.

————. "The Endocrine Role of the Thymus and Its Hormone, Thymosin, in Host Immunological Competence." Presented at National Foundation–March of Dimes conference, Harbor Springs, Mich., 1975.

————. "Nature and Biological Activities of Thymus Hormones—Prospects for the Future." Presented at New York Academy of Sciences, 1974.

————, and Goldstein, Allan L. "Is the Thymus an Endocrine Gland? Old Problem, New Data." *Perspectives in Biology and Medicine,* Spring 1968.

Whitten, Joan M. "Cell Death During Early Morphogenesis: Parallels between Insect Limb and Vertebrate Limb Development." *Science,* March 28, 1969.

Wilkes, Mahlon. Personal conversations.

Williams, Bernard. "The Makropoulos Case: Reflections on the Tedium of Immortality." In *Problems of the Self.* Cambridge: Cambridge University Press, 1973.

Williamson, A. R., and Askonas, B. A. "Senescence of an Antibody-forming Cell Clone." *Nature,* Aug. 11, 1972.

Willoughby, David P. "Animal Ages." *Natural History,* Dec. 1969.

Winter, Ruth. *Ageless Aging.* New York: Crown Publishers, 1973.

Wolf, Stewart. Personal conversations.

Woollcott, Joan. "The Mortal Cell." *Medical Affairs,* Sept. 1967.

Wright, Woodring E., and Hayflick, Leonard. "Contributions of Cytoplasmic Factors to In Vitro Cellular Senescence." *Federation Proceedings,* Jan. 1975.

————. "Enucleation of Cultured Human Cells." *Proceedings of the Society for Experimental Biology and Medicine,* Nov. 1973.

————. "Formation of Anucleate and Multinucleate Cells in Normal and SV40 Transformed WI-38 by Cytochalasin B." *Experimental Cell Research,* Vol. 74, 1972.

————. "Nuclear Control of Cellular Aging Demonstrated by Hybridization of Anucleate and Whole Cultured Normal Human Fibro-blasts." Prepublication manuscript.

Yanofsky, Charles, Cox, Edward C., and Horn, Virginia. "The Unusual Mutagenic Specificity of an *E. coli* Mutator Gene." *Proceedings of the National Academy of Science,* Vol. 55, 1966.

Yarborough, Donald. Personal conversations.

Yen, Samuel S. C. "Hypothalamic-Pituitary Discharge." *Reproductive Endocrinology,* 1973.

Young, Peter. "161 Years Old and Going Strong." *Life,* Sept. 16, 1966.

Young, Vernon R., Steffee, William P., et al. "Total Human Body Protein Synthesis in Relation to Protein Requirements at Various Ages." *Nature,* Jan. 17, 1975.

Yuncker, Barbara. "Is Aging Necessary?" (a series). *New York Post,* Nov. 18–22, 1963.

Index

i

A NOTE ON THE TYPE

The text of this book was set on the Linotype in a face called
Times Roman, designed by Stanley Morison for *The Times* (London)
and first introduced by that newspaper in 1932.
Among typographers and designers of the twentieth century,
Stanley Morison has been a strong forming influence,
as a typographical adviser to the English Monotype Corporation,
as a director of two distinguished English publishing houses
and as a writer of sensibility, erudition, and keen practical sense.

Composed by American Book–Stratford Press,
Brattleboro, Vermont
Printed and bound by Haddon Craftsmen,
Scranton, Pennsylvania